COPC Depression and Anxiety Intervention Guide

COPC Depression and Anxiety Intervention Guide

Richard Freeman, Chris Shearin, Stephen Gillam & Diane Plamping

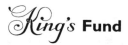

Published by
King's Fund Publishing
11–13 Cavendish Square
London W1M 0AN

© King's Fund 1997

First published 1997

ISBN 1 85717 124 1

A CIP catalogue record for this book is available from the British Library

Distributed by Grantham Book Services Limited
Isaac Newton Way
Alma Park Industrial Estate
GRANTHAM
Lincolnshire
NG31 9SD
Tel: 01476 541 080
Fax: 01476 541 061

Cover illustration by Clare Youngs

Contents

Preface

The purpose of this publication is to support primary care and community-based teams in seeking to develop their services for people with mental health problems. It is designed to make material about effective interventions accessible to every member of the team. The authors have adopted a distinctive approach, based on a community-oriented primary care (COPC) framework, to bring together material which is already available from many sources. The benefits of this approach arise from its action orientation.

The King's Fund Primary Care Group has produced a series of publications to support its COPC programme. The COPC approach was introduced in a step-by-step guide entitled *Community-Oriented Primary Care – A resource for developers*.[1] This publication is one of a series designed to help local teams as they work through the COPC framework. It reviews the evidence on anxiety and depression for primary health care teams who wish to plan a mental health intervention.

The need for material on mental health to support work within the COPC framework was identified in the initial programme evaluation. Several COPC pilot practice teams identified mental health as an important topic but one which the teams felt they lacked information on effective interventions for their practice populations.

To meet this need for decision support, the King's Fund convened an expert multidisciplinary steering group. The work was part funded by the NHSE North Thames Regional Office. This steering group decided to prioritise anxiety and depression from the wide agenda of mental health issues experienced in primary care. With their help we have drawn together the evidence on anxiety, depression, suicide and parasuicide which relates to general and community-based practice.

We would like to acknowledge the members of the steering group who have directed us towards the literature and have helped to shape this guide from concept to reality:

---

1. King's Fund 1994.

Janet Brotchie, Andrew Clark, Graham Curtis-Jenkins, Chris Dowrick, Hugh Freeman, Gyles Glover, Kevin Gournay, Keith Lloyd, Felicity Miles, Huw Richards, Allan Scott, Greg Wilkinson.

We would also like to thank all those who helped by reading and commenting on the earlier drafts of the document:

Elizabeth Armstrong, David Baldwin, Celia Boyes, Debbie Carter, Jack Fairbrother, Pat Jones, Michael King, David Lyon, Richard Maxwell, Frank Smith, Andree Tylee.

We also wish to thank North Thames Region and Ealing, Hammersmith and Hounslow Commissioning Agency for their support in field testing this material.

King's Fund Primary Care Group
February 1997

Chapter 1

Introduction

1.1 Purpose

This guide has been written for members of primary health care teams
(PHCTs) where the team has decided to run a community-oriented
primary care (COPC) programme on depression or anxiety. (If you are not
familiar with the COPC concept, this is explained in more detail in section
1.2.) The guide assumes that the team has completed its community
diagnosis and, through the prioritising stage, has chosen a mental health
intervention. At the next two stages, detailed problem assessment and
intervention planning, the team needs to establish practical interventions
that will work in a primary care environment. This guide is designed to
assist at those two stages.

The guide aims to help PHCTs develop more effective interventions in
depression and anxiety by following a COPC approach. As a result of
using this guide, PHCTs should:

- become aware of the range of proven primary care interventions for
  depression and anxiety;
- be able to select appropriate interventions for their situation
  ('appropriate' includes taking account of team skills);
- know where they can find out more about each intervention;
- be able to develop a practical plan for implementation of a chosen
  intervention.

Issues

The issues covered in this guide include:

- why depression and anxiety are appropriate for COPC intervention;
- which interventions are relevant for the two conditions;
- the main sources of information on interventions for depression and
  anxiety;
- the practical implementation of those interventions within a primary
  health care (PHC) setting.

We should stress, though, that this guide is not intended as the sole source of help for PHCTs when planning an intervention. In particular, they should always seek the specialist help available from or via their health commission, health authority or joint commissioning authority (JCA).

We also assume that the team has been trained in COPC methodology and has access to a copy of *Community-Oriented Primary Care: A Resource for Developers*.[2]

1.2 What is COPC?

COPC is an approach which seeks to promote better health through the strategic use of primary care resources. Through early identification of health problems, it seeks to offer interventions that will promote health and prevent further illness. COPC is one way of trying to use available resources to greater effect.

COPC has been defined as 'a continuous process by which PHC is provided to a defined community on the basis of its assessed health needs by the planned integration of public health with PC practice'.[3] While the focus of primary health care is usually the individual patient, with COPC the focus is the *community*. Thus, a COPC depression or anxiety programme will be aimed not only at those patients who are under treatment for depression or anxiety, but also at (a) those depressed or anxious patients who have not been diagnosed, and (b) those at high risk for depression and anxiety.

The stages in a COPC programme are illustrated in Figure 1.

The community diagnosis phase involves reviewing the health problems of the community. During the prioritising phase, the PHCT decides which health problem it wishes to work on. This guide assumes that the team has chosen depression or anxiety as its priority problem. In the detailed problem assessment phase, the team analyses the community's depression/anxiety problem in detail. At this point the team needs to find effective interventions which will enable it to address the problem. This is called intervention planning and the topic of this guide is *intervention planning for depression and anxiety*.

---

2. King's Fund 1994.
3. King's Fund 1994.

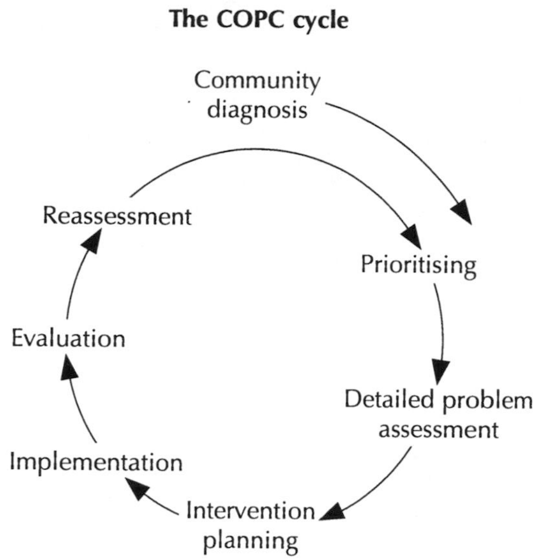

The COPC cycle

Figure 1 The COPC cycle[4]

1.3 Who the guide is for

When a PHCT plans a COPC intervention, it usually shares out the planning tasks. Collecting detailed information on the proposed intervention is just one of the tasks which might be delegated to any individual or group in the team. We hope therefore that any PHCT member will find this guide useful.

Above all, we have assumed your team has a commitment in principle to a mental health intervention. We have also assumed that you are searching for practical advice on how to intervene and do not need persuading of the benefits of intervention. The specific case for mental health interventions has already been set out in *The Health of the Nation*.[5]

1.4 Contents

We cover three areas in the guide:

- major depression;
- anxiety;
- suicide and deliberate self-harm.

---

4. King's Fund 1994.
5. *The Health of the Nation*, 1991.

These conditions have been selected because:

- they are widespread;
- they are under-diagnosed in primary care;
- the best place to detect them is primary care;
- they are responsive to primary care interventions, although less so in the case of suicide.

Some might argue that this guide should consider long-term mentally ill people, given the serious nature of their problems. While acknowledging the importance of care for this group, we have chosen to concentrate on depression and anxiety because:

- depression and anxiety are prevalent;
- between them, they take up far more practice time than do psychoses.

1.5 Opportunities for prevention

COPC programmes only make sense in circumstances where an at-risk group can be identified and where an intervention is available. Thus the first four questions that need to be asked are:

1   Is it possible to identify groups which are at risk of depression, anxiety and suicide?
2   Once we have identified the groups, can we identify those who need help?
3   For those who need help, are proven primary care interventions available?
4   Are interventions for depression and anxiety a good use of resources?

The rest of this section looks at these four issues at a general level. The remainder of the guide addresses the first three at a more detailed level for depression, anxiety and suicide in turn.

Prevalence

Knowing the prevalence of an illness helps in the planning of COPC programmes in two ways. First, an illness with a high prevalence is likely to yield large enough groups to make an intervention programme worthwhile. Second, comparisons of prevalence on a practice list with that in other similar locations can help to reveal under-diagnosis in a practice.

Psychiatric morbidity is widespread. Its estimated period prevalence rates are shown in Table 1. From this table it can be seen that about a quarter of those attending a surgery experience some psychiatric morbidity in any one year but that only about half of this is diagnosed. This table illustrates the widespread nature of psychiatric morbidity and its under-diagnosis. Primary care is well placed to identify and treat much of this illness.

Table 1 Period prevalence rates for psychiatric morbidity[6]

Setting	Period prevalence (n/1000 risk/year)
Community	260–315
Primary care (total)	230
Primary care (diagnosed)	101.5
Secondary care	20.8
Admissions	3.8–6.7

Since this guide is about depression, anxiety and suicide, we are particularly concerned with the prevalence for these problems. First, though, what are depression and anxiety?

Definitions

Major depression can be defined as 'a continuum of phenomena from a normal mood which is common and affects everyone from time to time to a severe disorder. A central feature of all depressive conditions is the lowering of mood, which when more severe may be accompanied by tearfulness and lack of ability to take interest in or pleasure from one's usual activities.'[7]

Anxiety is a normal response to stress or threat in daily life. Without it, people tend to become lethargic and to under-perform. However, when anxiety grows to the point where it interferes with daily life, it has then become a clinical problem. The essential characteristic of clinical anxiety is that it is out of proportion to the threat to the patient or too prolonged.

Depression and anxiety form a major part of psychiatric morbidity. The figures for major depression are shown in Table 2.

6. Paykel and Priest 1992, p 1198.
7. Paykel and Priest 1992, p 1198.

Table 2 Relative risk of depression[8]

Major depression aspect	Frequency
Depressed at any one time	5 in 100
Treated by GPs in a year	3 in 100
Referred to a psychiatrist	3 in 1000
Mild attack in lifetime	30 in 100

When anxiety is included in the picture, the prevalence is much greater, with around 30 per cent of people in the UK experiencing symptoms of depression or anxiety at any one time.[9]

The widespread nature of depression and anxiety, combined with their under-diagnosis, suggests that COPC may be a suitable approach to the problem. The next question to ask, then, is: 'Can we detect depression and anxiety at the primary care level?'

Opportunities to detect in primary care

The opportunities to detect depression and anxiety in primary care are strong for two principal reasons:

- patients who are aware that they have emotional problems have a strong tendency to consult their GPs;
- patients who have emotional problems but are not aware of them are still very likely to consult their GPs, but about a physical illness.

We now look at these two diagnostic opportunities in more detail.

The tendency to consult

There is wide-ranging evidence that those suffering from depression and anxiety see their GPs as the first source of help. For example:

- 15–30 per cent of GP consultations concern a mental health problem (20.4 per cent in the WHO study[10]);

---

8. Defeat Depression Campaign (nd).
9. Huppert *et al.* 1987.
10. Üstün and Sartorius 1995, p 372.

- when people were asked who they would consult if they suffered from depression, 60 per cent said they would consult their GP first. The next highest rating was 16 per cent for 'spouse';[11]
- 42 per cent of people over 35 who kill themselves consult their GP in the month before their suicide. For under 35s, though, consultation, at 10 per cent, is no higher than for all patients;[12]
- 70–90 per cent of people who develop a mental disorder will consult their GP within one year of the onset of the disorder, although they may not mention that disorder.[13]

This evidence suggests that primary care is uniquely well placed to detect depression and anxiety. Although patients may consult others (family, friends, social workers, religious workers, etc.), they overwhelmingly regard their GP as the person most likely to be able to help. One has to balance this, though, with the fact that many people do not think that their GP will be sympathetic.[14]

The overlap with physical illness

Many patients have both physical and mental symptoms. This is known as 'co-morbidity'. High levels of co-morbidity offer primary care an opportunity to detect depression and anxiety following the self-report of somatic conditions. Co-morbidity in adolescents is around 40 per cent,[15] while up to 50 per cent of general practice attenders may have some depressive symptoms.[16]

Patients with both a physical and a psychological illness are more likely to consult their GP than if they only have a psychiatric problem. Consultation rates for the former group can be nearly double those for the latter.[17]

While co-morbidity offers an opportunity to detect depression and anxiety, it also represents a problem in that the symptoms of the physical illness tend to mask those of the mental condition. This contributes to the under-

---

11. Defeat Depression Campaign 1992.
12. Vassilas and Morgan 1993.
13. van den Brink et al. 1991.
14. Defeat Depression Campaign 1992.
15. Smeeton 1992.
16. Effective Health Care 1993, p 2.
17. Vázquez-Barquero et al. 1992.

detection of the two conditions. GPs are three times more likely to miss major depression in patients with minor physical illness and five times more likely to miss depression in those with serious physical illness.[18] There is a double benefit in treating these patients, since chronic somatisers (i.e. patients who regularly complain about physical symptoms which are linked to their depression) who are really depressed may reduce attendances if the depression is treated.[19]

Value of intervention at primary care level

The case for intervention

It is natural to ask: 'Are we not doing all that we can already?' and 'Perhaps we just have to accept the current levels of depression and anxiety'. While this may be true for particular practices, overall the evidence suggests that the systematic tackling of depression and anxiety can yield appreciable gains. In a Swedish study where additional educational support was provided to GPs, the diagnosis and treatment of mental disorders significantly improved. In the year following the three-year programme researchers found that:

- the number of days spent in hospital by those with depressive disorders had decreased to 30 per cent of the expected days;
- suicide rates were significantly lower than for the control period and for Sweden as a whole;
- GPs identified more patients with depressive disorders and treated them more accurately;
- the prescription of major tranquillisers, sedatives and hypnotics declined.[20]

Other workers, though, have queried whether the reduction in suicides was due to the education programme or merely coincidental. If the effects were due to the education programme, then the later deterioration in the population suggests that such programmes need to be repeated at regular intervals.

---

18. Tylee AT *et al.* 1993.
19. Bass 1994.
20. Rutz *et al.* 1992.

The case for early intervention

While depression and anxiety often eventually go away, about half will persist without treatment.[21] One study of patients with neurotic disorders found that, after 11 years, 'a large proportion had become chronically unwell high users of primary care services'. The authors suggest that the findings support the need for early and effective treatment of such patients.[22]

For the duration of the morbidity, patients, and those around them, can experience a great deal of suffering and life-problems. Shortening the intensity and duration of the illness brings benefit to patients, their families, the health service and society. Primary care is well placed to deliver this benefit because:

- patients turn to primary care professionals for help (as discussed above);
- early detection may improve prognosis;[23]
- most patients with depression improve after treatment;
- depression which is recognised by a GP has a shorter duration than unrecognised depression, irrespective of the treatment offered.[24]

Interventions aimed at early detection offer a good use of resources, since they pre-empt the costs of the extra care needed if the cases were to become more entrenched. For these reasons primary care should aim for:

- early detection;
- the prevention of worsening of the condition;
- the prevention of relapse.

This is not to reject the need to intervene with patients whose condition has gone undetected for a lengthy period.

The costs of non-prevention

The costs of not intervening over depression and anxiety are considerable and have three consequences:

---

21. van den Brink *et al.* 1992.
22. Lloyd, Jenkins and Mann 1996.
23. Scott, Eccleston and Boys 1992.
24. Paykel and Priest 1992, p 1200.

- repercussions for the individual;
- costs to the health service;
- costs to society.

Consequences for the individual

There is substantial evidence that depression is a major source of undiagnosed morbidity. For example, depression causes as much suffering as chronic physical conditions such as arthritis.[25, 26] The burdens for the sufferer include:

- loss of daily functioning;
- loss of sense of well-being;
- untreated depressive illness becomes less responsive to treatment;
- depression is the commonest mental disorder in people who kill themselves.

These effects also impact on the families and friends of the patient. In total, they represent a substantial loss of quality of life for many people. Interventions that prevent or reduce depression and anxiety in patients can yield worthwhile gains for them and those around them.

Risks and costs for the health service

There are also considerable costs to the health service arising from depression and anxiety, including the following.

- First, there are the direct costs of the morbidity. In a typical GP list of 2000 patients, it has been estimated that 440 will be identified as at risk for depression according to the General Health Questionnaire (GHQ), and that the additional costs of these patients will be around £60,000 per year.[27]
- Second, there are the costs which arise from failure to treat the morbidity. Untreated depressive illness becomes more expensive to treat because of the increased risk of other problems such as suicide, deliberate self-harm, occupational problems, marital problems and accidents.

---

25 Eisenberg 1992.
26 Eisenberg 1992.
27 Lloyd and Jenkins 1995a.

- Third, there are the consequential costs to the health service as others develop morbidity caused solely or partly by the depressed patient's condition. For example, children of parents with depressive symptoms experience more emotional and cognitive problems. [28]

These costs are high. One aim of early intervention is to reduce them, either by preventing the onset of depression or anxiety, or by minimising its duration.

Risks and costs for others
Depression and anxiety have costs for society at large. For example:

- in 1991, working days lost through mental illness cost UK industry £6200m. Together with associated benefits costs, the total came to 1.3 per cent of gross domestic product. Half of the days lost were due to anxiety and stress and about a quarter to depressive disorders;[29]
- the total national cost of depression is estimated to be £3.5 bn per year. This includes health service costs and working days lost.[30]

Identifying those at risk

None of the above would be of much interest for COPC programmes if it were not possible to identify at-risk groups and, within those groups, to identify those in need of treatment. The practicalities of these two points are discussed below.

Primary prevention
At the primary prevention stage, a PHCT needs to know who is at risk. These individuals or groups can then be monitored in order to prevent or intercept the onset of anxiety or depression. Some of this monitoring may already be taking place in an informal manner. For example, all PHCT staff should be aware that mothers are at risk of post-natal depression. Hence, staff need to be extra watchful around post-partum so as to pre-empt the onset of depression. Health visitors are in a particularly good position to identify at-risk mothers.

---

28. Lloyd and Jenkins 1995b.
29. Thompson D 1993, p 39.
30. Defeat Depression Campaign (nd). *Questions and answers.*

In general, people with two types of life experience are likely to suffer depression and anxiety:

- those with acute or chronic stressors, such as housing, marriage and employment problems;
- those with life event problems, such as bereavement, divorce and children leaving home.

These groups are large and cannot be surveyed in detail on a continuing basis. If resources are to be used efficiently, then PHCTs will wish to identify those individuals within each group who are particularly vulnerable. A number of simple strategies are available for this, such as the Exeter Depression Audit. Not all the bereaved or all the unemployed become depressed. One of the key predictors for succumbing to depression is low self-esteem and a pessimistic attitude to life.

Secondary prevention

In secondary prevention the emphasis is on early detection because:

- cases detected early respond more readily to treatment;
- early detection reduces the distress suffered by patients and those around them.

There is also evidence that continued surveillance of patients is important. For example, one study[31] found that GPs reviewed the cases of those with chronic mental illness less frequently than they reviewed those with chronic physical illness. The authors developed a structured questionnaire to help GPs assess these cases more regularly. This led to increases in changes of treatment and of referrals.

1.6 Summary

The four basic requirements for a COPC intervention are met by depression and anxiety:

1   We know the risk factors for depression, anxiety and suicide. These may help in identifying groups for surveillance.

---

31. Kendrick, Burns and Freeling 1995.

2   We can identify, to varying extents, within those groups those who need help.
3   There are proven primary care interventions for depression and anxiety.
4   Prevention of depression and anxiety, along with their early detection, can mean efficient use of resources.

We now go on to look at depression, anxiety and suicide in more detail and explore the extent to which these four points hold.

Chapter 2

Depression

2.1 What is depression?

Sadness or worry sufficient to affect daily activities is experienced by 60–70 per cent of adults at some time.[32] In the more precise clinical sense, major depression is still common with, for western industrialised nations, a point prevalence of 2.3–3.2 per cent for men and 4.5-9.3 per cent for women and a lifetime risk of 7–12 per cent for men and 20–25 per cent for women. This makes depression a major concern for primary care teams and a good *potential* candidate for a COPC programme. However, effective interventions must be available before we can confirm that COPC potential. These will be explored in this section.

Depression is characterised by a wide range of behaviours, including those listed in Table 3.

Table 3 Behaviours in major depression[33]

Type of change	Examples
Emotional changes	A general feeling that life is not worth living, e.g. hopelessness and sadness
Cognitive changes	A lack of self-worth and a loss of confidence, e.g. self-hate, suicidal tendencies
Motivational changes	A loss of interest in life, e.g. apathy, fatigue, inability to concentrate
Neurovegetative symptoms	A general disruption and slowing down of daily life, e.g. disturbed sleep, poor appetite, loss of sexual interest

Classification by severity

There are many ways to classify depression. From a treatment point of view, the severity of the depression is a useful classification. The two main types are **major depression** (which can be mild, moderate or severe) and **dysthymia**

---

32. *Effective Health Care* 1993, p 2.
33. Goldberg, Benjamin, Creed 1994, pp 197–8.

Table 4 Severity of depression and treatment[34]

Severity	Diagnosis	Characteristics	Treatment
Mild	Adjustment disorder	Mild depressive symptoms for at least two weeks, following a stressful event (e.g. loss of a close relationship)	Cognitive behaviour therapy (CBT)
			Counselling (possibly)
			Possibly drugs
	Dysthymic disorder	Depression lasting at least two years, in which a pessimistic, negative outlook becomes an ingrained part of the person	CBT
			Counselling (possibly)
			Possibly drugs
Moderate	Major depression	An overwhelming depressed mood with significant sleep and appetite disturbances, including weight loss	Drugs
			CBT
Severe	Major depression with melancholia	Pervasive, stultifying depression with total loss of interest or pleasure, marked psychomotor retardation and early morning awakening	Drugs
			CBT

(chronic depression, present over a long period). This classification is useful because treatment is broadly dependent on severity, as shown in Table 4.

Criteria for major depression

The first stage in intervention planning is to identify the criteria for intervention.

No single symptom or behaviour confirms depression in a patient. The only way to diagnose depression is by the patient's accumulation of a range of symptoms and behaviours. The more symptoms the patient displays, the more likely that the diagnosis is depression. One of the sets of criteria is shown in Table 5. If a patient shows five of the symptoms, including one of depressed mood or diminished interest or pleasure, it is likely that the patient is suffering from major depression.

34. Columns 1–3 based on American Psychiatric Association 1987.

Table 5 Summary of DSMIII-R criteria for major depression.[35]

At least five of the following symptoms present during the same two-week period. This must include at least one of the symptoms *depressed mood* or *diminished interest or pleasure.*

1   Depressed mood
2   Markedly diminished interest or pleasure in normal activities
3   Significant weight loss or gain (if not on a diet)
4   Insomnia or hypersomnia
5   Agitated or retarded
6   Fatigue or energy loss
7   Feelings of worthlessness or excessive guilt
8   Diminished ability to think or concentrate, or indecisiveness
9   Recurrent thoughts of death or suicidal thoughts/activities

Other features of depression

- Usually begins in mid-20s and 30s, although it becomes more common with increasing age.
- Symptoms develop over days to weeks.
- 75 per cent of those who experience an episode will experience another.
- After an episode, patients may remain symptom-free for several years.
- For some, episodes become increasingly frequent.
- Untreated episodes may last from 6 to 24 months.
- Two-thirds of cases remit completely.[36]

Precipitants

Any one of a number of factors can precipitate depression in an individual. Some of these are listed in Table 6. However, none of these factors alone is enough to produce depression. The depressed state seems to occur in patients who feel helpless and pessimistic. Such patients generalise from negative experiences, so generating a feeling of hopelessness.

35. American Psychiatric Association 1987.
36. Depression Guideline Panel 1993, p 23.

Table 6 Precipitants of depression

- External stress (e.g. job loss, poor housing, relationship problems, bereavement, childbirth)
- Having relatives with depression
- Those physical diseases which precipitate depression (e.g. influenza)
- Physical illness in general, especially if chronic, painful, disabling or life-threatening

Prognosis

About a quarter of patients experience one attack only.

About half of patients experience a second attack after 2–5 years and, for some, the attacks continue to occur, particularly in old age.[37]

Patients with depression usually recover in the community, provided they experience the appropriate type of support or change in their lives. However, the prospects for recovery depend on the nature of the depression, as is illustrated in Table 7.

Table 7 Prognoses for types of depression[38]

Type	Prognosis
Following a severe loss event; patient otherwise has stable personality	Good recovery prospects
Depression associated with chronic adverse social or interpersonal circumstances	Poor recovery prospects
	Social and community interventions will be needed to attack the underlying problem
Depression associated with an abnormal personality	Poor recovery prospects
	Long-term support may be needed

Spontaneous recovery may arise from one or more of four changes listed in Table 8.

---

37. Wilkinson 1989, p 2.
38. Based on Goldberg, Benjamin and Creed 1994, p 203.

Table 8 Sources of spontaneous recovery

Type of change	Examples
Life events	Cessation of the stressful events or the occurrence of fresh-start events (e.g. a new job or better housing) aids remission
Social support	If the patient receives appropriate support from family, friends or elsewhere, remission is aided
Physical change	If the patient recovers from physical illness, this can aid remission
Natural remission	Unexplained remission may occur

None of this, though, should be used to argue against intervention. Untreated depression is a source of misery to the patient and affects the ability to function fully at work and in bringing up children. Also, for some, untreated depression can have serious consequences, including suicide.

Associated conditions

In many cases, the patient's depression is associated with some other condition, especially with chronic, painful, disabling and life-threatening conditions such as chronic arthritis, deafness, visual impairment or terminal illness, as shown in Figure 2.

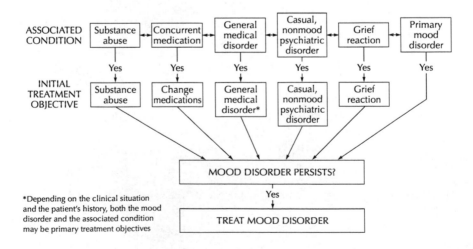

*Depending on the clinical situation and the patient's history, both the mood disorder and the associated condition may be primary treatment objectives

Figure 2 Conditions associated with mood symptoms[39]

39. Livingstone *et al.* 1990.

The figure illustrates the steps that need to be taken when there is an associated condition:

- first (top line of boxes in the figure): the associated condition is identified
- second (second line of boxes in the figure): a specific treatment for the associated condition is planned and implemented
- third (third and fourth lines of boxes in the figure): if the mood disorder is still present after the associated condition has been treated, then treat the mood disorder.

Where there is an associated condition, the doctor has to decide whether to treat both the depression and the associated condition as primary treatment objectives.

2.2 Who is at risk for depression?

Risk factors

In a COPC programme, the ability to identify at-risk groups can make the difference between a feasible and a non-feasible programme. In the case of depression, a number of at-risk groups can be identified. In some cases, the groups are easily identified (e.g. post-natal women); in others, it is questionable whether COPC methods could identify who was a member of the group (e.g. those who lack social support). A full range of risk groups is given in Table 9.

Table 9 Risk groups for depression

- Those with a prior episode of depression
- Those with a family history of depression
- Elderly people: 16 per cent have pervasive symptoms of depression[40]
- Post-natal women: up to 22 per cent develop depression[41]
- Inadequate child care following the loss of a parent (parental loss alone does not seem to pre-dispose depression)
- Poor parenting
- Those sexually abused in childhood[42]
- Those with experience of any kind of social trauma

40. Livingstone *et al*. 1990.
41. Richards 1990.
42. Hooper 1990.

There are also a number of circumstances which are associated with depression, including those listed in Table 10.

Table 10 Factors associated with depression

- Social disadvantage (e.g. unemployed people or those in poor housing)[43]
- A lack of social support
- Minority status[44]

But who will succumb?

The lists in Tables 9 and 10 can include a high proportion of patients in some practices so it helps to be able to identify who within these groups is particularly at risk.

An individual's depression may be caused by one of three types of factor:

- **predisposing factors** which increase vulnerability to a particular illness in the future
- **precipitating factors** which determine when the illness starts
- **maintaining factors** which prolong an illness and delay recovery.

Each of the three factors may be biological, social or psychological. Examples of these are given in Table 11.

Table 11 Causes of depression[45]

Type of cause	Biological examples	Social examples	Psychological examples
Predisposing	Genetic	Emotional deprivation in childhood	Poor parental role models
	Intrauterine damage		
		Bereavement	Learned helplessness
Precipitating	Recent infection	Recent life events such as unemployment or separation	Inappropriate response to a precipitating factor
	Malignant disease		

cont.

---

43. Gabe and Williams 1987; Lowry 1990.
44. Kessler and Neighbours 1986.
45. Jenkins *et al.* 1992, pp 12–14.

Table 11 cont.

Type of cause	Biological examples	Social examples	Psychological examples
Maintaining	Chronic pain	Chronic social stress, e.g. poor housing	Low self-esteem
	Loss of sensory ability, e.g. loss of sight		Doubts about recovering

In practice, people are protected by one set of factors and undermined by another. These undermining factors are called 'vulnerability' by Goldberg and Huxley. Figure 3 shows how the two sets of factors work to determine a person's condition.

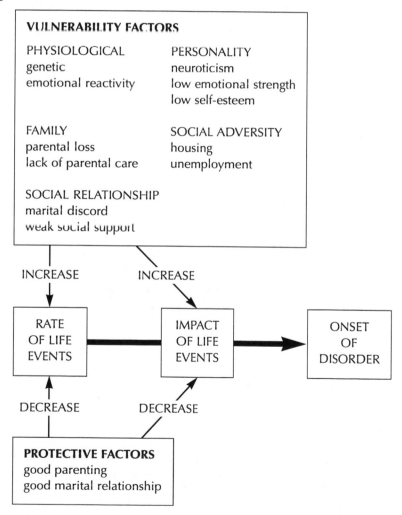

Figure 3 The relationship of vulnerability factors to one another [46]

46. Goldberg and Huxley 1992, p101.

Since COPC programmes need clear-cut rules or tests to identify members of the programme group, the practicality of using some of these factors to define groups is questionable. For example, a COPC group of post-natal women is easy to identify, since existing records will help determine which patients fall into the group. On the other hand, a COPC group of 'those who lack social support' would be hard to identify. Finding a rule or method to decide who was and who was not a member of that group would be difficult.

Special groups

Pregnant mothers

Pregnancy is a high-risk period for depression. Those mothers who are more likely to suffer depression during pregnancy and up to one year after include those with:[47]

- a past psychiatric history;[48]
- poor social support;[49]
- poor marital relationship;
- financial problems;
- an unplanned pregnancy.

Health visitors are well placed to identify those at risk.

Ethnic minorities

It is not clear whether people from ethnic minorities in Britain experience different levels of psychiatric morbidity compared to white British patients. However, there is evidence of under-diagnosis in both male and female ethnic minorities.

The WHO study identified four factors which lead to differences in the perceived prevalence rates between different locations:

- differences in health beliefs and care-seeking behaviours;
- differences in health delivery styles;
- variations in facilities at the locations;
- cross-cultural variations in responses to diagnostic questions.[50]

47. Sharp 1992.
48. Cox and Holden 1994.
49. Brown and Harris 1978.
50. Üstün and Sartorius 1995, p 373.

It is likely that some minority ethnic groups may present their depression or anxiety in ways which lead to under-diagnosis. For example:

- South Asian patients are more likely to present somatic symptoms;
- Indian patients may be more agitated and show less motor retardation than some other cultures;
- some cultures are more likely than others to express guilt;
- cultures in which weight is not usually measured are unlikely to report weight loss.[51]

Interviewing patients in their own first language may reduce this problem.[52] Awareness of common modes of presentation in a given ethnic group is also important.

Different ethnic groups may also respond to treatment in different ways. For example, Japanese Americans seem to need lower doses of antidepressants. Cognitive therapies need to take account of the patient's culture.

2.3 Diagnosis of depression

Symptoms

Depression is characterised by wide-ranging, non-specific symptoms, many of which are normal reactions to everyday life. These symptoms become indicative of depression when they accumulate and when they become functionally disabling. There is an important difference between 'I felt miserable yesterday and 'I was so miserable yesterday that I never got out of bed'.

The symptoms for depression fall into four categories:

- mood (e.g. sadness, tension, weeping);
- thinking (e.g. apathy, sensitivity, worthlessness);
- drive (e.g. wish to escape, feeling of being in a rut);
- physical (e.g. tiredness, loss of appetite or sleep, inability to relax).[53]

---

51. Bhugra 1995.
52. Lloyd 1992.
53. Wilkinson 1989.

Patients with physical complaints

Many patients, though, present somatic symptoms. Such patients are characterised by repeated consultations for aches and pains, none of which proves significant.

Frequent attenders

Frequent attenders include many with psychiatric morbidity. One study found that 18 per cent of frequent attenders were diagnosed as having neurotic depression and 24 per cent as having an anxiety state.[54]

Diagnostic methods

Core features

One simple initial approach is to use the nine questions of the Defeat Depression Campaign card as shown in Table 12. By counting the 'yes' answers, the depression, if present, can be classified as mild, moderate or severe using the scoring system in Table 13.

Table 12 Diagnostic questions for depression[55]

If low mood, ask:	1 How bad is it? How long for?
	2 Have you lost interest in things?
	3 Are you more tired than usual?
If 'yes' to any of the above:	4 Have you lost confidence in yourself?
	5 Do you feel guilty about things?
	6 Do you find it difficult to concentrate?
	7 How are you sleeping?
	8 Have you lost appetite/weight?
	9 Do you feel life is not worth living anymore?

Table 13 Scoring the diagnostic answers from Table 11[56]

Score from Table 12	The depression is:
At least two from the first three *plus* two others	Mild
At least two from the first three *plus* three or four others and/or yes to No. 5	Moderate
Most of these in severe form and/or yes to Nos. 5 and 9	Severe

54. Karlsson, Lehtinen and Joukamaa 1995.
55. Armstrong and Lloyd 1993.
56. Armstrong and Lloyd 1993.

Another recently published approach is based on producing flipcards for each of the International Classification of Diseases (ICD)-10 PHC Chapter 5 categories. For example, the card for Depression (F32*) is shown in Figure 4.

Depression – F32*

Presenting complaints

May present initially with one or more physical symptoms (fatigue, pain). Further enquiry will reveal depression or loss of interest.

Sometimes presents as irritability.

Diagnostic features
LOW OR SAD MOOD
LOSS OF INTEREST OR PLEASURE

Associated symptoms are frequently present:

- disturbed sleep
- guilt or low self-worth
- fatigue or loss of energy
- poor concentration
- disturbed appetite
- suicidal thoughts or acts.

Movements and speech may be slowed, but may also appear agitated.

Symptoms of anxiety or nervousness are frequently also present.

Differential diagnosis
If hallucinations (hearing voices, seeing visions) or delusions (strange or unusual beliefs) are present, see also card on acute psychotic disorders F23* about management of these problems. If possible, consider consultation about management.

If history of manic episode (excitement, elevated mood, rapid speech) is present, see card on bipolar disorder F31*.

If heavy alcohol use is present, see cards on alcohol use disorders F10* and drug use disorders F10*.

Figure 4 Diagnostic card for depression[57]

---

57. Üstün *et al.* 1995, p 213.

1	2	3	4	5	6	7	8	9	10	11	12	13	14

RISK INDICATOR

NAME			DATE			
Bereavement Relationship	Yes	No	Male		Female	
Marital Problems Date of Divorce	Yes	No	Living Alone		Yes	No
Single Parent No of dependent children Recent Childbirth	Yes .... Yes	No No	Social Contacts: Supportive/Unsupportive			
Caring for Disabled Person Relationship .... Details: Any support?	Yes	No	Recent change of residence Yes No (e.g. new immigrant) Details:			
Physical Health: Any disabilities Sensory Physical Serious physical illness Details:			Employed/Unemployed How long? Difficulties at Work Details:		Yes	No
Family history Details: Medication:	Yes	No	Financial Problems Details:		Yes	No
Family Problems	Yes	No	Housing Problems Details:		Yes	No

Figure 5 Health risk assessment card [58]

A simple health risk assessment card is shown in Figure 5. This card is used to identify how many risk factors a patient has. That number of blocks is then highlighted across the top of the card to alert the GP to the patient's level of risk.

58. Armstrong 1995, p 92.

Rating scales

Self-administered rating scales are effective in identifying depression in primary care. They not only save staff time, but help doctors improve the accuracy of their diagnoses.[59,60] Where doctors were given additional training in using general health questionnaire (GHQ) data, diagnoses increased.[61]

These findings are important in the COPC context, since a COPC programme needs a reliable means of both establishing prevalence at the detailed problem assessment stage and of tracking changes in prevalence during the programme. Rating scales, given that in some cases they can be completed by patients, offer an economical method of collecting population data.

Beck depression inventory

This is a 21-question self-administered scale. It can be used to measure depression on a first visit and to monitor progress during treatment. The maximum score is 63; mild depression scores 14–20; moderate corresponds to 21–26; and severe to scores of over 26. The test is not suitable as a diagnostic tool.

General health questionnaire

The 12-point GHQ is not specifically designed for depression but can be a useful screening tool. It is self-completed and can be done in the surgery. The scale can be used as an audit tool in general practice.[62]

Edinburgh Post-Natal Depression Scale

Standard depression scales produce unreliable results when used with post-natal women. The Edinburgh Post-Natal Depression Scale overcomes this problem and is reliable and acceptable to patients.[63] A copy of the scale appears in Appendix 1.

59. Johnstone and Goldberg 1976.
60. Zung *et al.* 1983.
61. Rand *et al.* 1988.
62. Armstrong 1995, pp123–126.
63. Cox *et al.* 1987.

SDDS-PC

The Symptom Driven Diagnostic System for Primary Care (SDDS-PC) is a computerised system for diagnosing mental disorders. It has: a five-minute patient questionnaire; six five-minute diagnostic modules (which include one for major depression and one for generalised anxiety); and a longitudinal tracking form. This is a new system, first reported in 1995.[64]

The geriatric depression scale

This is a 30-item self-report questionnaire, requiring only Yes/No answers. Other versions exist, such as the 15-item one. A study to compare the usefulness of 15-, 10- and 4-item versions of the test found that all three alternatives worked well in place of the 30-item test. The reliability of the four-item version was found to be 'somewhat low', but the authors still felt it had merit in the busy surgery. The four questions were:

- Are you basically satisfied with your life?
- Have you dropped many of your activities and interests?
- Do you feel happy most of the time?
- Do you prefer to stay at home, rather than going out and doing new things?[65]

Diagnostic problems

Depression is persistently under-diagnosed, with only about 50 per cent of cases being recognised on first presentation. There are a number of circumstances which contribute to the missed diagnosis, including:

- the patient has a physical illness;
- the patient has mostly somatic complaints;
- the consultation time is short;
- the doctor lacks communication skills;
- the patient particularly emphasises tiredness rather than sadness or depression.[66]

---

64. Olfson *et al*. 1995.
65. van Marwijk *et al*. 1995.
66. Freeling, Rao and Paykel 1985; Bridges and Goldberg 1985; Davenport, Goldberg and Millar 1987; Dowrick 1992; Wright and Perini 1987; Tylee *et al*. 1993.

Generally, patients under-report depression and anxiety to doctors mentioning as few as 20–30 per cent of their emotional problems. Doctors may reinforce the patient's behaviour by seeming to concentrate on physical symptoms rather than asking questions about the patient's psychological and social life.[67] Doctors and patients can be said to collude in treating somatic conditions, so jointly avoiding the more sensitive area of distress.[68] However, other research suggests that patients do not mention their depression because they think doctors are not interested or are unable to help.[69] In a MORI poll, 60 per cent of people agreed with the statement 'people with depression feel embarrassed to consult their GP'; 51 per cent were concerned about their doctor's reaction, and 23 per cent felt their doctor would be irritated or annoyed by the consultation.[70]

Providing information to patients may make them more willing to seek treatment. The *Health of the Nation* programme includes a booklet which aims to educate people about mental illness and to encourage them to seek help.[71]

Life-threatening illnesses

People with life-threatening illnesses may display a different range of symptoms, so making depression more difficult to diagnose.[72]

Alcohol misuse

People with alcohol misuse are more likely to suffer psychiatric co-morbidity. Diagnosing the patient as alcohol-dependent can therefore help in identifying the psychiatric problem. One approach, the Primary Care Evaluation of Mental Disorders (PRIME-MD) diagnostic system, reported a 71 per cent increase in the detection of alcohol misuse.[73]

In the case of patients with alcohol dependence, their depression can be caused by the toxic effects of the alcohol. The depression may remit within two weeks of abstinence and detoxification.[74]

---

67. Good, Good and Cleary 1987.
68. Goldberg and Huxley 1992.
69. Dowrick 1994.
70. Defeat Depression Campaign 1992.
71. Department of Health 1995.
72. Saunders 1995.
73. Johnson *et al.* 1995.
74. Davidson 1995.

Elderly people

Depression in elderly people may well go undetected by primary care teams. One study of a complete community found that 16 per cent of those aged 65 years or over had an identifiable mental health condition, but only a proportion of these were being treated by their GPs. The number of patients receiving antidepressants was lower than the researchers expected.[75]

Since depression in elderly people can be masked by the normal effects of ageing, care is needed to detect signs that an elderly person may be suffering from depression. Such signs include:

- agitation;
- cessation of eating;
- forgetfulness;
- frequent attendance;
- mutism;
- poor concentration;
- self-neglect.[76]

Differential diagnosis

Differential diagnosis in depression involves: (a) determining that the patient does have the symptoms of depression; (b) checking for any other illness that may be the cause of that depression; and (c) eliminating physical causes of any somatic symptoms.

The following four-point checklist is helpful here:

1   Check for major depression;
2   Check for substance, alcohol misuse and current medications;
3   Check for biological causes or associates of the depression;
4   Check for other non-mood psychiatric conditions.[77]

Elderly people and dementia

It is possible to mis-diagnose a depressed elderly patient as having dementia. The guidelines in Table 14 help to distinguish the two conditions.

---

75. Mental Health Foundation 1995.
76. Royal College of Psychiatrists and Royal College of General Practitioners (nd), p 6 (adapted).
77. Depression Guidelines Panel 1993.

Table 14 Differential diagnosis of depression and dementia in elderly people [78]

Clinical features	Depression	Dementia
Onset	Relatively rapid	Insidious
Cognitive impairment	Fluctuating	Constant
Memory/comprehension	Will respond to treatment	Progressive deterioration/ little or no response to treatment
Sense of distress	Yes	No/blunting of feeling
Self-image	Negative	Unaffected
Somatic symptoms	Typical	Atypical except for sleep disturbance

2.4 Interventions for depression

Primary prevention

Primary prevention involves monitoring groups in which there is a greater occurrence of depression. These groups include:

- those with alcohol or drug problems;
- those with chronic, painful or life-threatening conditions;
- those with minority community status;
- people with visual or hearing impairment;
- post-natal mothers;
- those recently separated or divorced;
- bereaved people;
- elderly people;
- disabled people;
- socially isolated people;
- adults with a history of sexual or physical misuse in childhood.

However, monitoring such groups *en bloc* is costly. A more effective approach is to identify those who are (a) vulnerable and (b) approaching or experiencing a life event that might trigger depression. These individuals can be offered support to:

---

78. Wilkinson 1989.

- reduce vulnerability, e.g. through the use of cognitive therapy and problem-solving therapy;[79]
- reduce life difficulties, e.g. through social services;
- increase social support, e.g. through befriending services.[80]

In each case, the key to prevention is early referral to support and resources which may be outside the practice.

Social support

A variety of forms of social support have been found to be helpful. These include:

- Placing citizens' advice bureaux inside general practices can deliver effective support to those who have life problems. Apart from the referral to other sources of help, in one group of 150 attenders, 50 were helped to make benefit claims totalling over £50,000. Checks showed that these clients were additional to the bureau's work.[81]
- A computer program was used within a practice to help patients identify welfare benefits to which they were entitled. In this case, 22 per cent of those who used the program found they were entitled to further benefits.[82]

While both these approaches may seem marginal to the work of a general practice, for many, because of the link between poverty and ill health, improved material conditions are essential to reducing their vulnerability to depression.

Community links

In one project, an external facilitator helped practices acquire knowledge of local services available to support patients. These included: mental health teams, social services and voluntary agencies. The evaluation of this work has not yet been published.[83]

---

79. Myners-Wallis *et al.* 1995.
80. Jenkins *et al.* 1992, p 27.
81. Paris and Player 1993.
82. Gillam 1994.
83. Armstrong 1994.

Health promotion

In general, all forms of health promotion will assist in the primary prevention of depression and anxiety, since physical illness may exacerbate both conditions and *vice versa*.

Secondary and tertiary prevention

Early detection and treatment are the major form of secondary prevention. The methods available are discussed below under physical interventions, psychological interventions and social interventions. Each method is first discussed separately, and then the combining of methods is discussed.

One study found that intervention made no difference, prognosis being the same for detected and undetected cases.[84] It is possible that, in these case, GPs unconsciously selected the more protracted cases for treatment.

Psychological interventions

On the whole, psychological interventions aim to reduce patients' vulnerability by helping them to acquire new skills and understanding.

Problem-solving therapy
In problem-solving therapy, patients are taught how to solve problems. This involves learning to use a five-stage approach:

- adopt a problem orientation;
- define the problem in concrete terms;
- generate an exhaustive list of solutions;
- evaluate each solution and choose the best;
- implement the solution and monitor the outcome.[85]

Cognitive behaviour therapy
Cognitive behaviour therapy seeks to modify the patient's negative thoughts and behaviour without focusing on the underlying psychological causes of the problem. The method involves:[86, 87]

---

84. Dowrick and Buchan 1995.
85. Silver and Ruckle 1989, p 361.
86. King's Fund 1994.
87. France and Robson 1986.

1   A detailed analysis of the problem. This might involve the patient keeping a diary or someone observing the patient. The analysis aims to establish the patient's present behaviour patterns, answering questions like 'what does the patient do?', 'when does this occur?'.

2   A treatment plan based on small steps towards the treatment goal is negotiated. Patients usually record their own progress and are fully involved in reviewing and amending the treatment plan. The patient's friends and relatives may be involved in helping the patient implement the plan.

3   The plan may include the use of other techniques such as relaxation or control of hyperventilation. However, in a cognitive behaviour therapy programme, the main aim is to teach the patient new behaviour patterns and more appropriate thoughts.

CBT can produce a rapid improvement compared to 'treatment as usual', but it is unclear whether it is effective in the long term when used alone or with other treatments. [88]

Interpersonal therapy

This approach aims to resolve those interpersonal and social problems of the patient which worsen the depression. The process involves explaining the nature of the depression to the patient and reviewing the patient's relationships. It is particularly relevant where the depression has been precipitated by social or interpersonal problems, especially:

- abnormal grief reactions;
- interpersonal disputes (e.g. marital conflict);
- stressful role transitions or life changes;
- deficits in sustaining personal relationships (e.g. fears about intimacy). [89]

Overall, these forms of psychotherapy appear to be beneficial in three out of four cases. [90]

Counselling

Counselling provides support and reassurance while allowing patients to express their emotions and explore their problems. The process encourages

---

88. *Effective Health Care* 1993, p 6.
89. Silver and Ruckle 1989, p 359–360.
90. Free and Oei 1989; Nietzel, Russell, Hemmings and Gretter 1987; Smith and Glass 1977; Corney 1990.

the patient to talk through his or her problem and to identify and evaluate solutions for themselves, knowing that the counsellor is there to offer support.[91]

The effectiveness of counselling for the treatment of severe depression is not clear.[92] It appears to be more appropriate for people encountering a specific life event such as job loss, bereavement or relationship problems[93] and for those who need strong support such as the rootless, those suffering from loss of self-esteem and worth and 'heart-sink' patients (i.e. patients whose frequent visits make the doctor's heart sink). It seems likely that the more articulate are the best suited to counselling. However, the evidence for the effectiveness of counselling is patchy – and sometimes obscured by a lack of clarity about exactly who was being treated. Generally, CBT may be preferable.

When comparing the effectiveness of counselling against referral to clinical psychologists, allowance needs to be made for the fact that counsellors and psychologists tend to see different patients. Counsellors tend to see more patients with anxiety, depression, marital problems, child management and physical illness. Psychologists, on the other hand, tend to see more patients with relationship problems and personality disorders.[94]

In considering whether to use counselling, its public acceptance might be relevant. Eighty-five per cent of the public rate counselling very or fairly effective in treating depression, while the figures for anti-depressants and tranquillisers were 46 per cent and 40 per cent. These figures were little different for the sub-group of those who had suffered from depression.[95] Overall, though, it might be concluded that 'whether or not counselling is effective is a fundamental question that still needs to have a definitive answer'.[96]

Social interventions

Individual social interventions
Social interventions (such as social learning therapy) aim to help the

---

91. Sheldon 1992.
92. *Effective Health Care* 1993, p 7.
93. Irving and Health 1989.
94. Burton, Sadgrove and Selwyn 1995.
95. Defeat Depression Campaign. 1992.
96. Armstrong 1995, p 48.

patient remove structural difficulties and reconnect with family and society. The interventions may be task-oriented and focus on empowerment. Methods include:

- helping the patient build relationships;
- helping the patient become an active member of the community;
- helping the patient get a new job or training;
- helping the patient find better housing;
- helping the patient gain access to resources, e.g. respite care.

Such support is best given by whichever PHCT member has the opportunity to build a continuing relationship with the patient – for example, a health visitor for a woman with post-natal depression. Sometimes, a social worker is well placed for this approach.

The effectiveness of social support seems to be limited, although it can be effective with women experiencing an acute episode on top of a long-standing depression. [97] It is important, though, only to use the approach where (a) the social problems are a clear cause of the depression and (b) those problems can be ameliorated.

Group social interventions
Group support systems are often used to help women suffering from post-natal depression. These are usually run by health visitors. A number of factors seem to help in the success of these groups, including:

- avoiding referring to post-natal depression in the name of the group, e.g. a name such as 'mothers support group' might be used;
- complete confidentiality so that the women are prepared to talk openly about their problems without fear of being referred for other treatment;
- rolling membership so that mothers do not have to wait to join a group;
- weekly sessions over anything from six to fifteen weeks;
- active listening skills on the part of the group leaders. [98, 99, 100, 101, 102]

---

97. *Effective Health Care* 1993.
98. Pitts 1995.
99. McClarey and Stokoe 1995.
100. Painter 1995.
101. Foyster 1995.
102. Jones, Watts and Romain 1995.

Another approach has been to use more formal teaching with groups of mothers, teaching such things as coping mechanisms and communications skills. [103] One group which was based on non-aerobic exercises rated the opportunity for discussion more highly than the exercise or the relaxation sessions. [104]

Physical interventions – drugs

In treating depression, drugs are important in providing symptom relief, in shortening the period of depression and in preventing relapse.

The drugs available to treat depression include tricyclic and related antidepressants, monoamine oxidase inhibitors and selective serotonin reuptake inhibitors (SSRIs). [105]

When using SSRIs and the tricyclic and related antidepressants, factors to be considered include: [106]

- they are effective for major depression;
- amitriptyline produces about 70 per cent improvement;
- tricyclics affect reaction time (e.g. driving or using machinery);
- low dose regimes are less effective and may not be superior to placebos;
- relapse is a common problem but treatment for four-to-six months (and longer for relapse and recurrences) after the episode has resolved will reduce relapse.

When using SSRIs, factors to be considered include: [107]

- they are more expensive than older tricyclics;
- they are less toxic in overdose than some of the older tricyclics and are safe with alcohol;
- their efficacy is similar to tricyclics;
- patient acceptability (as measured by drop-out) may be better than for tricyclics;
- tolerability is better than for older tricyclics, but new tricyclics are well-tolerated;

103. Eastwood 1995.
104. May 1995.
105. Mead 1995.
106. *Effective Health Care* 1993, p 4.
107. *Effective Health Care* 1993, pp 5–6.

- amitriptyline and clomipramine are tolerated noticeably less well than SSRIs.

All antidepressant drug treatments have problems associated with compliance and patient understanding of the nature of the drugs. Patients say that they are not given enough information on the side-effects, or on what the drugs are for. It has been found that treatment with antidepressants:

- suffers from poor patient compliance; this is partly because the drugs can be slow to act and may give rise to side-effects before benefits;
- requires careful negotiation with the patient to ensure that drugs are the best treatment option and there is a good chance of patient compliance;[108]
- may appear economical in its use of GP time but regular monitoring of side-effects and compliance is an unavoidable add-on cost;
- needs to take account of apparent patient confusion of antidepressants with tranquillisers which patients see as addictive. In a national study, 78 per cent of respondents thought antidepressants were addictive. In the same study, 91 per cent of respondents thought that people suffering from depression should be offered counselling but only 16 per cent thought they should be offered antidepressants. Further, one reason why patients are reluctant to consult GPs is the view held by 58 per cent of the sample that 'GPs tend to give just pills'; 59 per cent of those who had suffered from depression supported this statement.[109]

This clearly demonstrates that, if drugs are prescribed, care must be taken to establish the patient's acceptance of such treatment. In a parallel survey of doctors, the majority said they would initiate drug treatment for a depressed patient.[110]

Finally, whenever drugs are used, prolonged treatment (typically six months) is essential.

How do we choose which one to use?
The key determinant in whether to use drugs is the severity of the depression. Otherwise, there is little to choose between antidepressants for efficacy in

---

108. Ley 1988.
109. Defeat Depression Campaign 1992.
110. Royal College of Psychiatrists 1992.

treating symptoms: all provide effective relief, but antidepressants differ in their side-effects and costs. In prescribing, the main points to consider are:

- at doses of 125–150 mg daily tricyclic antidepressants are effective in patients in general practice with depressive illness;
- there is no evidence that doses of 75 mg daily or lower are effective, although SSRIs are effective above daily doses of 20 mg;
- antidepressants are effective in depressive disorders satisfying the criteria for major depressive disorders and in episodes a little below this threshold;
- antidepressants are effective even in the presence of life stresses;
- after successful treatment, drugs should be administered for a further four to six months to prevent relapse.[111]

How do we choose which treatment to use?

Depression only

The choice of treatment depends on the nature and severity of the depression. Typically, this will be a combination of drugs and some other treatment. With four or more symptoms, antidepressants are essential. Table 15 summarises treatment guidelines.

Table 15 Treatment guidelines for depression[112]

General nature of the depression	Intervention to consider
Effects of early deprivation	Psychodynamic therapy
Unrewarding lifestyle	Social and behavioural change
Negative thinking	Cognitive therapy and psychotherapy
Major depression	Cognitive therapy and psychotherapy
	Drug treatments appear to be the most effective

Cost and patient acceptability will also need to be considered.

Depression and other psychiatric disorders

Where the patient has depression and some other psychiatric disorder, a more complex set of treatment decisions has to be made. The US

111. Paykel and Priest 1992, p 1200.
112. Wilkinson 1989 (adapted).

Department of Health has summarised the treatment decisions as shown in Figure 6.

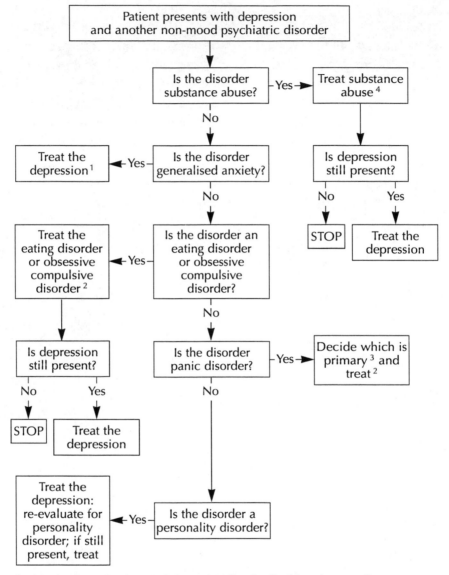

¹ When the depression is treated, the anxiety disorder should resolve as well.

² Choose medications known to be effective for both the depression and the other psychiatric disorder.

³ Primary is the most severe, the longest standing by history, or the one that runs in the patient's family.

⁴ In certain cases (based on history), both major depression and substance abuse may require simultaneous treatment.

Figure 6 Treatment decisions for depression accompanied with other psychiatric disorders [113]

113. Depression Guideline Panel 1993, p 44.

Depression and other physical illness

Similarly, where the patient has depression and some other physical illness, a more complex set of treatment decisions has to be made. The US Department of Health has summarised these treatment decisions as shown in Figure 7.

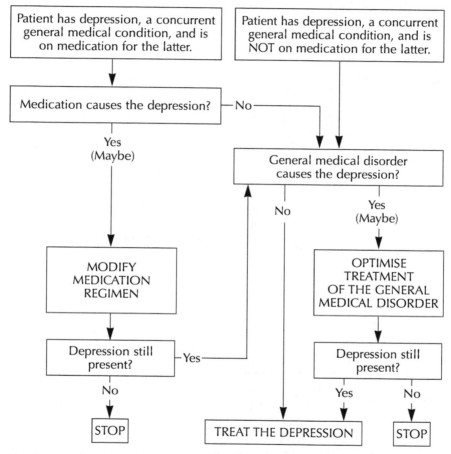

Note: In some clinical situations, treatment of the depression (e.g. if severe, incapacitating, or life-threatening) cannot be delayed until treatment for the general medical disorder has been optimised.

Figure 7 Treatment decisions for depression accompanied with other physical illness[114]

Particular care is needed in treating and supporting the patient with a life-threatening physical illness. Not only is there a need to deal with the physical symptoms, but also to help the patient develop a fighting spirit, reinforcing their genuine hopes and maintaining open communication.[115]

114. Depression Guideline Panel 1993, p 57.
115. Saunders 1995.

Summary of treatments

A general summary

The guidelines for the general management of depression based on the new classification of mental disorders are given in Figure 8. The authors note that 'modifications to reflect local conditions can be made during translation or adaptation of these cards'.[116]

Essential information for patient and family

1   Depression is common, and effective treatments are available.
2   **Depression is not a weakness or laziness**; patients are trying their hardest.

Specific counselling to patient and family

1   **Ask about risk of suicide.** Can the patient be sure of not acting on suicidal ideas? Close supervision by family or friends may be needed.
2   Plan short-term **activities which give enjoyment or build confidence.**
3   **Resist pessimism and self-criticism.** Do not act on pessimistic ideas (for example, ending marriage, leaving job). Do not concentrate on negative or guilty thoughts.
4   If physical symptoms are present, **discuss link between physical symptoms and mood** (see card on unexplained somatic complaints). [not reproduced here]
5   After improvement, discuss signs of relapse, plan with patient action to be taken if signs of relapse occur.

Medication

1   **Consider antidepressant drugs if sad mood or loss of interest is prominent for at least two weeks and four or more of the following symptoms are present:**
    - Fatigue or loss of energy
    - Guilt or self-reproach
    - Thoughts of death or suicide
    - Agitation *or* slowing down of movement and speech
    - Disturbed sleep
    - Poor concentration
    - Disturbed appetite

If good response to one drug in the past, use that again.

If older or medically ill, use newer medication with fewer side-effects.

If anxious or unable to sleep, use a more sedating drug.

cont.

Figure 8 Management card for depression[117]

---

116. Üstün *et al.* 1995, p 213–214.
117. Üstün *et al.* 1995, p 212.

Figure 8 *cont.*

Medication

2   **Build up to effective dose** (for example, imipramine starting at 25–50 mg each night and increasing to 100–150 mg in 10 days) – lower doses if older or medically ill.

3   **Explain how medication should be used**

Medication must be taken every day.

Improvement will build over 2–3 weeks.

Mild side-effects may occur and usually fade in 7–10 days.

Check with the doctor before stopping medication.

4   **Continue antidepressant** drugs for at least 3 months after symptoms improve.

Specialist consultation

1   If **suicide risk** is severe, consider consultation and hospitalisation.

2   If **significant depression persists**, consider consultation about other therapies.

3   **More intensive psychotherapies** (for example cognitive therapy, interpersonal therapy) may be useful for acute treatment and relapse prevention.

An audit summary

When auditing the treatment of depression, the criteria in Table 16 and Table 17 have been suggested. Table 16 lists those aspects of treatment for which there is firm research evidence. Table 17 lists those aspects for which there is some evidence to support their effectiveness.

Table 16 'Must do' audit criteria for the treatment of depression[118]

- The records show that the diagnosis of depression is correct
- The records show that, at diagnosis, the patient has been assessed for risk of suicide
- Patients with major depression are treated with antidepressants and/or cognitive therapy
- Antidepressants must be prescribed in therapeutic doses
- Drug treatment should be continued for at least four months after the episode of depression has resolved

118. Eli Lilley Centre, Leicester (nd), p 3.

Table 17 'Should do' audit criteria for the treatment of depression[119]

- After commencement of treatment the patient should be reviewed within three weeks, and the risk of suicide re-assessed
- Patients who have responded fully in the acute phase of treatment are seen at least once every month during the maintenance of treatment

Other approaches to audit have been suggested.[120]

GP training

There is evidence that GPs find depression an unrewarding area to work in and that their attitudes to depression differ from those of psychiatrists. This might suggest that educational programmes for GPs need to be matched to their attitudes and beliefs.[121]

A number of studies have showed the benefits of training GPs in the detection and treatment of depression. One approach which aimed to 'increase understanding among practice staff and health professionals working in the wider community' used training sessions with the whole of the practice staff, including community nurses and receptionists. All the participating practices found the process so useful that they wished to continue it.[122] Training GPs in the use of a structured questionnaire to assess chronic mental patients also brought beneficial results.[123]

One study used a programme of patient education, GP education and psychiatric care to treat depression. Each patient had two initial study sessions, one with the GP and one with a psychiatrist. Educational material (a booklet and a video) was given to the patient. This process aimed to motivate patients to take an active role in their own treatment. Each participating GP had had a half-day training session. The treatment then used a structure process of two visits to the GP (visits 1 and 3) and two to the psychiatrist (visits 2 and 4). The programme achieved improvements in patient adherence to antidepressant usage, and both patients and GPs found it helpful.[124]

---

119. Eli Lilley Centre, Leicester (nd), p 3.
120. For example, the Appendix of Armstrong 1995.
121. Kerr, Blizard and Mann 1995.
122. Williams 1996.
123. Kendrick, Burns and Freeling 1995.
124. Katon *et al.* 1995.

Practice nurse role

Armstrong describes a three-stage model of how practice nurses could be involved in mental health, emphasising that what can be done in reality depends on the time the nursing staff have and their skills. The model is summarised in Table 18.

Table 18 A model for practice nurse involvement in mental health[125]

Stage	Key elements
1 Health assessments	This stage involves the practice nurses assessing patients' mental state whenever they make any health assessment. Armstrong provides a set of guidelines for this (page 116).
2 Monitoring and supporting	Typical activities might be: • monitoring antidepressant use • mental health promotion incorporated into other work • liaising with Accident and Emergency over those at risk of suicide • supporting anxious patients
3 Specialist roles	Typical activities might be: • assessment of depressed patients • supporting patients withdrawing from tranquillisers • mental health audit

The role of the community psychiatric nurse in depression

The wide range of treatment methods for depression inevitably draws in a wide range of staff roles. The role of the CPN has particularly come under discussion with the increasing use of CPNs in counselling. Recent work has shown that this does not save GP time and deflects CPNs from work with more serious health problems where their skills are particularly needed, including:

• behaviour therapy (where the CPN is trained for this);
• psychosocial interventions with chronic schizophrenics and their families;
• case managers for those with serious and acute mental illness.[126]

---

125. Armstrong 1995.
126. Gournay and Brooking 1994.

There seems to be a particular role for the mental health nurse in the treatment of manic depression, where the nurse can be involved in:

- the assessment of suicide risk;
- supporting self-management;
- educating people about the Manic Depression Fellowship (a self-help organisation);
- supporting carers.[127]

Social worker role in depression

Social workers fall into two types: (a) those generically qualified; and (b) those qualified as approved social workers (ASWs).

The generically qualified will have skills in working with adults and will be able to assess family and community situations and to provide general support.

ASWs are trained in risk assessment and in compulsory admission procedures. They are well qualified to assist in preventing hospital admission, discharge planning and in negotiating care plans.

2.5 Monitoring and evaluating depression

At the individual level

Once a patient has recovered, regular monitoring is necessary at about monthly intervals for a six-month period. Patients should be encouraged to monitor themselves for any return of symptoms and to report these to the doctor when they occur.

Each consultation should be recorded in a standard format so that the progress of the depression can be monitored. A practice protocol can be developed for this based on the Burton and Freeling model.

The regular assessment of patients with chronic mental illness can be assisted by the use of a structured questionnaire.[128]

---

127. Hill and Shepherd 1996.
128. Kendrick, Burns and Freeling 1995.

At the population level

A number of aspects of the practice can be audited to help gather a population view, as shown in Table 19.

Table 19 Audit measures for a population view

Measure	Practical detail
Comparisons of recorded and expected prevalence	These can be broken down by patient group (particularly the high-risk groups discussed above) to check for under-detection with particular patient groups.
Extent of use (and change of use) of different therapies	Each of the different treatments can be monitored: • drug use • therapies use • counselling use. Measures of use might include: • length of period of treatment • cost of treatment.
Effects of an intervention	A number of indicators could be monitored to detect the effects of a depression intervention, including: • more cases detected (i.e. recorded and expected prevalence come more into line) • shorter depression episodes • reduced chronic depression • less time off work • changes in referral rate to psychiatrists, psychologists, psychotherapists and counsellors.

It is likely that referral rates will increase at first and then decline. Increased *detection* skills, but inexperience of treatment strategies will lead to greater involvement of secondary care services. Subsequently, increased confidence in *treatment* skills will lead to a decline in referrals to psychiatrists.

Changes in general health following a depression intervention may not be demonstrable at the practice level. Where data can be aggregated over a larger area, the effect may be measurable.

Chapter 3

Anxiety

3.1 What is anxiety?

Anxiety is a normal response to stress or threat in daily life. Without it, people tend to become lethargic and to under-perform. However, when anxiety grows to the point where it interferes with daily life, it has then become a clinical problem. The essential characteristic of clinical anxiety is that it is out of proportion to the threat to the patient or too prolonged. A patient's negative thinking is often key to intensifying their reaction to the threat and so precipitating anxiety.

The symptoms of anxiety are of four types:

1   cognitive (e.g. negative thinking);
2   physical (e.g. palpitations);
3   emotional (e.g. hypersensitivity);
4   behavioural (irritability, sleep pattern disturbance, difficulty in making decisions).

It can be hard to distinguish between depression and anxiety because there is an overlap in symptoms and the two conditions can occur together or follow one another.

Prevalence

Clinical anxiety is a fairly widespread condition. Its estimated prevalence is:

• men: 2–4 per cent
• women: 3–4.5 per cent.

However, anxiety among patients attending a GP's surgery is likely to be commoner since the onset of any illness produces clinical anxiety in 10 per cent of patients.[129]

---

129. Goldberg, Benjamin, Creed 1994.

Anxiety rarely starts over the age of 40. It is a common presenting symptom for new episodes of depression.

Types of anxiety

There are a variety of forms of anxiety. These are set out in Table 20. This guide concentrates on the commonest forms: generalised anxiety, phobias and panic disorder.

Table 20 Types of anxiety

Type of anxiety	Main characteristics
Generalised anxiety	Persistent and generalised state of anxiety, not associated with any particular situation
Phobias	An intense need to avoid certain situations or objects
Panic disorder	A sudden onset of anxiety or panic accompanied by an intense need to avoid a particular situation or object
Obsessive compulsive disorder	A strong compulsion to think or behave in a certain way which the patient feels is wrong but cannot resist
Post-traumatic stress disorder	An intense reaction to a profoundly distressing experience (e.g. a major accident), usually involving the patient's repeated reliving of the experience

Causes of anxiety

The causes of anxiety fall into two categories: patient background and patient experience.

Patient background

- Some patients have a genetic predisposition to anxiety.
- Some personality types are predisposed to anxiety.

Patient experience

- Stressful events may trigger the onset of clinical anxiety (such events, of course, always trigger anxiety).

- Some patients seem to become anxious through conditioning – they learn their anxiety. This may well occur in their upbringing.
- Panic disorders can be associated with disturbed childhoods, although, often, no obvious association is found.
- Agoraphobia can be associated with traumatic childhood events, although again, often, no obvious association is found.[130]
- Patients who dwell on their symptoms of normal anxiety may invoke clinical anxiety.
- Poor parenting.

Most people do not suffer anxiety when they experience these sort of events. Those who do are said to be vulnerable.[131]

The single most important factor shared by all patients with anxiety is that the patient has learnt an inappropriate response to a situation or series of situations, or even to life itself. **The fact that anxiety is learnt has an important bearing on its treatment which needs to focus on learning new responses.**

3.2 Who is at risk for anxiety?

Risk factors

The risk factors for anxiety are a mix of patient experience and patient vulnerability to that experience.

Experience risk factors include:

- **chronic stressors**, e.g. housing problems, relationship problems and employment difficulties
- **major life events**, e.g. divorce, bereavement, job loss and children leaving home.

Vulnerability risk factors (i.e. ones which increase the stressful impact of the experience factors) include:

- lack of a confiding/warm/loving relationship;
- a lack of a sense of self-worth;
- a sense of hopelessness;

---

130. Faravelli *et al.* 1985.
131. Goldberg and Huxley 1992.

- poor time management;
- lack of self-assertiveness;
- lack of leisure interests or hobbies;
- inability to relax.

Groups/types exposed to the risk factors

While specific groups are more likely to develop, or be diagnosed as having, clinical anxiety (e.g. women and those under 40), it may be more helpful to identify groups who (a) are experiencing the relevant stressors, and (b) seem to fall into the vulnerable category, that is, who have the personality type for anxiety. Thus, from a COPC programme point of view, the at-risk groups might be the ones in Table 21, but identifying the vulnerable within the groups is essential.

Table 21 Potential COPC groups for anxiety disorders

Those with:

- housing problems
- relationship problems
- employment difficulties

and those experiencing:

- divorce
- bereavement
- job loss
- children leaving home.

3.3 Diagnosing anxiety

The initial diagnosis is concerned with deciding whether the patient is suffering from anxiety at all. Then the diagnosis can concentrate on distinguishing between cases of:

- mild anxiety;
- phobia;
- severe anxiety.

Symptoms

The symptoms of anxiety fall into four main categories, as illustrated in Table 22.

Table 22 Categories of symptoms of anxiety

Type of symptom	Examples
Cognitive symptoms	Negative thinking
Physical symptoms	Palpitations, tachycardia, sweating, tremors, lumps in the throat, restlessness, easily tired
Emotional symptoms	Hypersensitivity
Behavioural symptoms	Irritability, sleep pattern disturbance, difficulty in making decisions, poor concentration

Anxiety questions

Table 23 illustrates a short set of questions for diagnosing generalised anxiety. If the patient answers 'yes' to two or more of the first four questions, then the second set of questions are asked also. Using a score of one point for each 'yes' answer, a total score of five or more indicates a 50 per cent chance of clinical anxiety. This anxiety question scale can be administered by any trained member of the PHCT and used as an initial screening device in a COPC programme. It could, for example, be used at the detailed problem assessment stage to establish the current population prevalence of anxiety.

Table 23 Generalised anxiety question scale[132]

Questions to ask the patient

- Have you felt keyed-up/on edge?
- Have you been worrying a lot?
- Have you been irritable?
- Have you had difficulty relaxing?

If 'yes' to two of the above, go on to ask:

- Have you been sleeping poorly?
- Have you had any of the following: trembling; tingling; dizzy spells; sweating; frequency; diarrhoea?
- Have you been worried about your health?
- Have you had difficulty falling asleep?

Score one point for each 'yes'. Add up the score. Five or more indicates a 50 per cent chance of a clinically important disorder.

---

132. Goldberg *et al.* 1994 (adapted).

Once the initial diagnosis of anxiety has been made, the more specific symptoms of each type of anxiety can be looked for.

General anxiety

Specific symptoms:

- complaints of anxiety, worry or tenseness; and
- at least three of the general symptoms (Table 23).

The more of the general symptoms the patient shows, the greater the probability that the diagnosis should be anxiety.

Panic attacks

Specific symptoms:

- the patient may report feelings of sudden panic or dread – when no other symptoms are present, this is a panic attack;
- the attacks are recurrent;
- have both cognitive and psychological components, e.g. dread and tachycardia;
- no other symptoms (unless there are complications such as panic disorder with agoraphobia).

Phobias

Specific symptoms:

- the patient's anxiety may only occur under specific conditions (for example, in the open or in the presence of certain animals) – these are the symptoms of a phobia;
- a recurrent avoidance of a specific situation or object/class of objects;
- fear of that situation;
- patient awareness that the fear is irrational: 'I can't explain why, doctor'.

A phobia is also characterised by its seriously disabling nature which distinguishes it from a mere distaste of a situation, e.g. many people dislike spiders; only a phobic patient is disabled by this reaction.

Diagnostic methods

About half of the cases of depression and anxiety are not initially recognised by doctors. Patients may contribute to the non-diagnosis through preferring to talk about physical rather than emotional symptoms. Thus, the patient prefers to talk about his/her headaches than to tell the doctor that his/her spouse walked out last week. To overcome this problem, doctors can adopt an interviewing style which makes it easier for the patient to talk about his/her emotional problems.

The approach combines an open, relaxed questioning style with encouraging the patient to talk about his/her feelings. For example, if the patient says, 'I seem to be having a lot of headaches lately', a suitably open response from the doctor would be, 'Tell me why you think that is'.

Table 24 summarises the recommended style. In some cases, though, just listening will prove to be the sole intervention that is needed.

Table 24 Interview style to encourage patients to talk about their emotional problems[133]

At the start of the interview:

- makes eye contact with the patient
- is able to clarify the complaint

General interview skills:

- picks up verbal clues
- picks up non-verbal clues
- can deal with over-talkativeness
- deals well with interruptions
- isn't buried in the notes
- adopts less avoidant, more relaxed posture
- makes facilitatory noises while listening
- is less urgent and hurried
- doesn't give information early

cont.

---

133. Goldberg and Huxley 1992 (adapted).

Table 24 *cont.*

Types of question:

- asks directive questions about psychiatric symptoms, e.g. 'How are you sleeping?'
- asks closed questions about psychiatric symptoms, e.g. 'Have you had difficulty falling asleep?'
- makes supportive comments
- asks about home.

Screening

Practice screening may be of two types. First, the practice may screen high-risk groups as a matter of course. Second, it may select specific groups for a COPC programme. Typical groups for screening are:

- post-natal women;
- people over 75;
- unemployed people;
- new patients.

(These same groups could be screened for depression.)

Rating scales

A number of anxiety rating scales are available. A general measure of anxiety is provided by the *State Trait Anxiety Inventory* (Spielberger) and by the *Anxiety Checklist* (Beck).

A more comprehensive scale with an emphasis on phobias is the *Marks and Matthews Fear Questionnaire* (see Appendix 2).

Differential diagnosis

The anxiety/depression distinction

We have mentioned the difficulty of distinguishing between depression and anxiety. Table 25 lists symptoms which are more typical of depression than anxiety. If these symptoms predominate, a diagnosis of depression should be considered.

Table 25 Symptoms more typical of depressive than anxiety conditions[134]

- Lowered mood
- Loss of interest
- Thoughts of guilt or worthlessness
- Loss of energy
- Fatigue
- Early morning wakening
- Broken sleep
- Indecision
- Inability to concentrate
- Somatic symptoms
- Loss of appetite
- Loss of libido
- Suicidal ideas

Other psychiatric, physical or drug-related problems

There is also a need to consider other possible causes of the symptoms:

- is the anxiety linked to another psychiatric illness? (e.g. schizophrenia);
- is there physical illness? (e.g. endocrine problems);
- are drugs or alcohol involved?

Co-morbidity

Anxiety is increasingly seen in cases of co-morbidity. Using the diagnostic approaches above (including the scales, if necessary) can help to reveal the anxiety. This should then be treated alongside any other condition.

3.4 Interventions for anxiety

Primary prevention

We have mentioned the stressors that contribute to anxiety and the key influence of patient vulnerability. Primary prevention aims to reduce the problems faced by the patient and to increase the patient's capacity to face those problems. The methods include:

- promoting coping skills to overcome vulnerability;
- supporting vulnerable individuals at critical life events;
- offering support to at-risk individuals at life event times, e.g. childbirth, bereavement, divorce, job loss and relationship crises;

---

134. Wilkinson 1992a, p 15.

- promoting a healthy lifestyle [135] through advice on diet, exercise, smoking and alcohol;
- assisting patients' access to other services such as benefits and housing.

The precise mix for any one patient requires careful judgement. For example, a heavy smoker may gain more from problem-solving help than from advice to give up smoking.

Secondary and tertiary prevention

Physical interventions

Physical interventions play little part in the treatment of generalised anxiety; their limited role is discussed below.

Drug treatments

In most cases, no drug treatment should be offered. On the whole, the role of drugs in the treatment of anxiety is to facilitate the conditions under which other treatments can take effect. Drugs, therefore, tend to be used for the following:

- where there is also significant depression;
- to help the patient through a short-term problem, such as facing a much-feared operation;
- to give the patient the support to relearn appropriate behaviour, e.g. agoraphobics may be prescribed drugs to keep at hand when relearning to venture out of the home. The knowledge that they have the drugs handy helps them overcome the fear of how to cope with a panic attack;
- to help break the vicious circle where the cause of the anxiety has been removed and, effectively, the patient is anxious about being anxious. If other treatments have failed at this point, drugs can be used to relieve the symptoms for a short period while other treatments continue. The aim, though, still remains to teach the patient new behaviour patterns and the drug treatment is used solely to facilitate this;
- when the symptoms are so severe that the patient suffers a serious disruption to social and work life;
- in particular anxiety disorders, such as panic disorder and obsessive compulsive disorder.

135. Lloyd and Jenkins 1994.

There are three key risks in using drugs:

- dependency, particularly with benzodiazepines (antidepressants, though, are not addictive);
- masking the condition and so delaying the introduction of a full treatment programme. Relearning is key to anxiety treatment and the longer the anxiety state exists, the harder it is to treat;
- they reinforce the idea that anxiety is predominantly a medical condition so the patient does not take responsibility for changing his/her understanding and behaviour.

Benzodiazepine withdrawal

Where benzodiazepines have been prescribed, the problems of withdrawing these from patients can arise. Withdrawal symptoms include anxiety, depression, loss of appetite, perspiration and perceptual disturbance.[136] The PHCT should have a protocol for withdrawal from benzodiazepine use.[137]

Psychological interventions

Psychological intervention starts with the GP's examination of the patient, especially if the patient fears that he or she has a physical illness. In examining the patient:

- acknowledge the source of anxiety or pain – do not deny the patient's symptoms;
- explain to the patient that he/she has no physical illness – do not convey any doubt to the patient who will only use this to confirm his/her anxious state: 'I knew that doctor would not find out what was really wrong with me';
- explain to the patient that he/she is suffering from anxiety, that this is common, real and can be treated;
- explain to the patient how his/her condition has arisen, i.e. that the patient has learnt to respond to certain stresses or situations in an inappropriate way and that it is possible to learn a new way of responding – you may well be able to point to a time when the patient did not react inappropriately and so reinforce the fact that the patient has learnt to become anxious;

---

136. Wilkinson 1992a, p 43.
137. For example, Wilkinson 1992a, p 44.

- reassure the patient that members of the PHCT can help and explain what help is available and how and when you will organise it;
- if the patient expects a drug to be prescribed, explain to the patient why this would not help.

Advice

Patients suffering from anxiety need plentiful advice, help, support and reassurance. Advice will probably not be used on its own but may, for example, be part of counselling or relaxation.

Many members of the PHCT team are in a good position to offer advice. With suitable training and a practice protocol, the adviser can be whoever is most trusted or works most with a particular patient. As well as the doctor, the CPN, PN, HV, counsellor and SW are well placed to support patients with advice and reassurance.

Printed advice sheets can be used alongside other treatments and probably work best when the sheet is explained to the patient at the time it is given out. [138, 139] An example sheet appears in Appendix 3. [140]

Relaxation

Most patients with symptoms of anxiety will benefit from being able to relax more. Telling them to relax may make matters worse: 'Now I have to worry that I am not learning to relax'. Such patients should be advised about the availability and benefits of attending relaxation classes. These include activities such as yoga, meditation, autogenic training and hypnosis. If a COPC programme is being planned, the team should consider whether it makes sense to offer relaxation classes on practice premises or to recommend those offered in the local community. The community diagnosis might have identified local classes but may not have established their suitability for the practice's patients. A check on who is running the classes and their qualifications is essential.

Relaxation tapes can also be recommended and copies might be kept in the practice for loan. If used, they can prove a less time-consuming intervention.

---

138. Milne and Covitz 1988.
139. Sorby *et al.* 1991.
140. France and Robson 1986, pp 63–66.

The recommendation of relaxation may well follow from the use of advice and support as an intervention.

Counselling

The value of counselling for anxious patients is still unclear. There have been some positive results but counselling is not a general solution.[141, 142] Despite this, counselling can be popular with patients, so PHCTs need to consider with care where they stand on counselling.

Where counselling is used, it seems important to bear in mind that:

- patients should be given a choice between counselling and some other treatment;
- thought should be given as to whether the individual patient is likely to benefit from counselling;
- as many PHCT members as is sensible should be trained in counselling so that the counselling builds on an existing trusted relationship; the training is lengthy;
- health workers with some counselling training (e.g. HVs) can be just as effective as full-time counsellors, especially in post-natal depression;[143]
- when the counselling is done by a GP, the time involved in anxiolytic treatment and counselling is about the same.

For those patients who do not respond to counselling, cognitive behaviour therapy (CBT) and problem-solving can be an effective treatment.

Cognitive behaviour therapy

The principles of this approach have already been discussed in the section on depression (see pp. 33–4). CBT can be used with patients suffering from generalised anxiety, phobias and panic attacks.

In the case of phobias, though, the additional aspect of graded exposure is involved. Here, the patient is gradually helped to tolerate the feared situation. For example, if the patient fears furry objects, the patient might first learn to accept being in the same room, but not near to, a cat. Gradually, the patient accepts closer and closer contact.

---

141. Corney R 1992, p 336.
142. Catalan *BMJ* 1984
143. Cox *et al.* 1987.

Cognitive behaviour therapy may appear time consuming but the literature suggests that it is not. Robson quotes interventions of 15–30 minutes with an average programme of treatment taking 2 hours 34 minutes per patient.[144] The more complex problems are likely to involve much more time.

Problem-solving

Problem-solving is a behaviour change therapy in which patients are helped to identify the cause of the anxiety and to agree a programme of actions to change their behaviour.[145, 146]

Four sessions of problem-solving can be effective for a wide range of anxiety and depression cases, producing reductions in PSE (present state examination) scores at 11 and 28 weeks. Patients show greater satisfaction with the problem-solving approach compared to controls who receive any other GP treatment.[147]

Problem-solving is normally carried out by a clinical psychologist, but the skills can be taught to PHCT staff where they are likely to make enough use of the investment.

Anxiety self-help groups

Self-help groups with professional support can be effective and acceptable to patients. These can mix a range of treatments such as information, problem-solving and relaxation. In one trial, patients attended eight one-and-a-half-hour sessions over an eight-week period. By the end of the sessions, one-third had stopped taking medication and around 20 per cent had reduced their dosage. Subsequently, patients made fewer visits to their GPs.[148]

Social and psychosocial interventions

Anxiety is often exacerbated by social and personal problems in a patient's life. Where the patient's problems are of this type, social workers and CPNs can help by:

- (sometimes) directly intervening to ameliorate the source of the problem;
- helping the patient recognise interpersonal problems and encouraging the patient to seek help with them;

144. Robson 1992.
145. King's Fund 1994.
146. France and Robson 1986.
147. Catalan *et al.* 1991.
148. Long and Bourne 1987.

- supporting the patient;
- assertiveness training;
- time management training.

How do you choose which interventions to use?

The overriding principles in the choice of a method or methods of treatment are:

- make sure that all the patient's problems have been identified through the assessment – if the patient has more than one problem (e.g. a physical and an emotional problem), then each must be treated;
- make sure that if drugs are used their main purpose is to enable other treatments to take effect;
- monitor the patient's progress carefully and adjust treatment as necessary – prolonged use of a treatment which is not working makes future interventions more difficult;
- ensure that the method(s) are acceptable to the patient.

The options are summarised in Table 26. This range of options would involve, according to the skills needed, GPs, psychologists, psychiatric nurses and social workers.

Table 26 Treatments for anxiety disorders[149]

Form of anxiety	Possible drugs	Other treatments
Generalised anxiety disorder	DiazepamBuspirone	Relaxation Cognitive therapy Anxiety management
Simple phobia		Desensitising by gradual exposure
Social phobia	Moclobemide Phenelzine Beta blockers	Anxiety management Cognitive therapy Social skills training
Panic disorders	Tricyclic or SSRIs Phenelzine Alprazolam	Cognitive therapy Anxiety management
Agoraphobia	Tricyclic or SSRIs	Desensitising by gradual exposure Cognitive therapy

149. Adapted from Wilkinson 1992.

3.5 Monitoring and evaluating anxiety

In a COPC programme, monitoring always has two functions:

- to provide data for clinical decisions about the patient;
- to provide data for population evaluation against the original detailed problem assessment.

This requires devising data collection formats which meet both needs.

Normally, monitoring for six months is sufficient. Thereafter patients should be encouraged to return if they feel they are becoming anxious again.

The regular assessment of patients with chronic mental illness can be assisted by the use of a structured questionnaire.[150]

---

150. Kendrick, Burns and Freeling 1995.

Chapter 4

Suicide and deliberate self-harm

4.1 Suicide and deliberate self-harm

Prevalence

There are about 4500 suicide deaths in the UK each year. Of these, about three-quarters are male suicides. Generally, suicides have fallen in recent years, but they are increasing in the 15–24 age group for men. Nine out of ten people who commit suicide suffer from mental illness.[151]

Around 15 per cent of diagnosed depressives will commit suicide and there are a further 100,000 deliberate self-harm (DSH) cases a year in the UK, i.e. about 3–4 patients per practice. These relatively low figures suggest that suicide and DSH *per se* are not ideal candidates for COPC programmes, since evaluating the effectiveness of the programme would be impractical at practice level. However, a depression COPC programme will have in its target group some of those who are prone to suicide so the points of this section would be relevant in that context.

Criteria for suicide and deliberate self-harm

Suicide

Suicide is self-destruction where there is evidence that the individual intended to kill himself or herself.

Deliberate self-harm

Deliberate self-harm involves intentional acts which the individual knows will result in personal injury.

4.2 Who is at risk of suicide and DSH?

Risk factors

Certain groups are at a much higher risk of suicide than the general

---

151. Thompson 1993, p 23.

population. For example, current/former psychiatric patients are ten times more likely to commit suicide, and drug misusers 20 times more likely.[152]

There are a number of factors which are associated with an increased risk of suicide. These are shown in Table 27. However, it is not possible to predict with any accuracy who will attempt suicide so it is problematic for a COPC type of intervention.

Table 27 Factors associated with increased suicidal risk[153]

Demographic and social

> Male – especially young males
> Over 45 years
> Separated, divorced or widowed
> Social isolation
> Unemployment
> Recent bereavement

Medical

> Severe or chronic physical illness
> Depressive illness
> Alcoholism
> Personality disorder
> Previous episode of self-harm

4.3 Identifying potential suicides

Symptoms

The only specific indicator of suicide is an expressed intention to commit suicide. This is reflected in the questions that are used in detecting potential suicides (see Table 28).

Recognition aims to identify those who have suicidal thoughts and to identify those who can be treated by the GP or need referring to secondary care.

---

152. Gunnell and Frankel 1994, p 1227.
153. Goldberg, Benjamin, Creed 1987, p 324 (adapted).

Table 28 Identifying potential suicides[154]

Patient ideas/intentions	Treatment
Patient has no:	• Treat depression
• suicidal ideas • suicidal intentions • suicidal plans • previous attempts at suicide	
Patient has:	1 Treat for depression 2 Monitor closely
• ideas present • intentions present	3 ?Refer
But no:	
• plans • history	
• Intentions present • Plans present • Has tried before	1 Refer urgently 2 Monitor closely 3 Treat depression

Clinical clues and associated conditions

Detecting potential suicides requires that they come into the surgery. Of those over 35 years, 26 per cent had seen their GP in the week before their suicide and 48 per cent in the four weeks before. Those under 35, though, were no more likely to have consulted their GP than non-suicidal patients.[155] However, of those in one of the highest risk groups, those with a previous psychiatric history, half had seen their GP in the 15 days prior to their suicide.[156]

Despite these guidelines, there is no reliable way to predict who will attempt suicide.[157] Surveillance and intervention are best focused on those in high-risk categories and particularly those with a previous history of attempts and/or a previous psychiatric history.

154. Armstrong and Lloyd (nd) (adapted).
155. Vassilas *et al*. 1993.
156. Matthews *et al*. 1994.
157. Goldstein RB *et al*. 1991.

4.4 Interventions for suicide and deliberate self-harm

Suicide

Given that 50 per cent of those who commit suicide have previously indicated their intention to a doctor, suicide is to some extent preventable. However, no specific intervention has been found to affect suicide rates apart from the work on GP education.[158] At best, steps can be taken to remove the means of suicide and to make help as accessible as possible. Steps which can be taken include:

- removing the means of self-harm (especially toxic drugs) from the patient;
- choosing antidepressants which appear relatively safe in overdose;[159]
- making the primary care services as accessible as possible so as to maximise the patient's opportunity to ask for help (even though the appeal may be oblique);
- educating the friends and relatives of the patient about the warning signs and the type of support they can give;
- appropriate management of chronic physical or depressive illness;
- assisting the patient to make contact with and use support agencies in the community, such as the Samaritans.

Although the list above includes removing toxic drugs, the specific role of antidepressants in suicide is less clear. Most depressed patients who commit suicide are not taking antidepressants at the time of death. This indicates that their deaths are more due to the failure to adhere to the medication than to its toxic effects.[160] Prevention should therefore include assisting the patient to keep taking antidepressants.

Deliberate self-harm

In general, the points made about potential suicides apply to deliberate self-harms as well. Additionally, the practice can:

- offer counselling to accident and emergency attenders since there is significant incidence of multiple attendance;

---

158. Rutz *et al.* 1992.
159. Freemantle *et al.* 1994.
160. Isacsson *et al.* 1994.

- identify vulnerable groups in general practice;
- make an urgent referral to secondary care if the level of risk is high.[161]

---

161. Fairbrother. Suggestions based on unpublished research. Private communication.

References

American Psychiatric Association 1987. Diagnostic and Statistical Manual of Mental Disorders. 3rd ed. *American Psychiatric Association*, Washington DC.

Armstrong E 1994. *The KCW FHSA: Mental health facilitator project*. St George's Hospital Medical School.

Armstrong E 1995. *Mental Health Issues in Primary Care*. Houndmills: Macmillan.

Armstrong E and Lloyd K 1993. Rational steps ease depression. *Practice Nurse* 1–14 Nov, pp 690–693.

Armstrong E, Lloyd K *et al.* (nd). *Management of Depression in Primary Care*. (Card). Defeat Depression Campaign.

Bass C 1994. Somatisation. In: Paykel E and Jenkins R (eds) *Prevention in Psychiatry*. London: Gaskell.

Bhugra D 1995 Depression and culture. *Practice Nurse* June, pp 507–510.

Bridges KW, Goldberg DP 1985. Somatic presentation of DSMIII psychiatric disorders in primary care. *Journal Psychosometric Research* 29, pp 563–569.

Brown GW and Harris TO 1978. *Social Origins of Depression*. London: Tavistock.

Burton and Freeling 1982. *Journal of Royal College of General Practitioners* 32, pp 558–561.

Burton MV, Sadgrove J and Selwyn E 1995. Do counsellors in general practice surgeries and clinical psychologists in the National Health Service see the same patients? *Journal of the Royal Society of Medicine* 88 (February), pp 97–102.

Catalan J, Gath D, Edmonds G and Annis J 1984. The effects of non-prescribing of anxiolytics in general practice: I Controlled evaluation of psychiatric and social outcome. *British Journal of Psychiatry*: 144; 593–602.

Catalan J, Gath D, Bond A and Martin P 1984. The effects of non-prescribing of anxiolytics in general practice: II Factors associated with outcome. *British Journal of Psychiatry*: 144; 603–610.

Catalan J, Gath DH, Bond A, Day A and Hall L 1991. Evaluation of a brief psychological treatment for emotional disorders in primary care. *Psychological Medicine*: 21; 1013–1018.

Corney R 1992. The effectiveness of counselling in general practice. *International Review of Psychiatry*; 4, No. 3/4, pp 331–337.

Corney RH 1990. Counselling in general practice: does it work? *Journal of the Royal Society Medicine* 83, pp 253–257.

Cox JL, Holden JM and Sagovsky R 1987. Detection of postnatal depression: development of the 10-item Edinburgh Postnatal Depression Scale. *British Journal of Psychiatry* 150, pp 782–786.

Davenport S, Goldberg D, Millar T 1987. How psychiatric disorders are missed during medical consultation. *Lancet* 1, pp 439–441.

Davidson KM 1995. Diagnosis of depression in alcohol dependence: changes in prevalence with drinking status. *British Journal of Psychiatry* 166, pp 199–204.

Defeat Depression Campaign 1992. *Attitudes towards depression*. MORI Poll for Defeat Depression Campaign.

Defeat Depression Campaign (nd). *Defeat depression: How common is it?* Defeat Depression Campaign press release.

Defeat Depression Campaign (nd). *Questions and answers*. The Royal College of Psychiatrists.

Department of Health 1995. *Mental Health: Towards a Better Understanding*. Department of Health.

Depression Guidelines Panel 1993. *Depression in Primary Care. Vol. 1 Detection and diagnosis*. US Department of Health and Human Resources.

Dowrick C 1992. Improving Mental Health Through Primary Care. *British Journal of General Practice* 42, pp 382–386.

Dowrick C 1992. Why do the O'Sheas consult so often? *Social Science Medicine* 34, pp 491–497.

Dowrick C 1994. Private communication.

Dowrick C and Buchan I 1995. Twelve-month outcome of depression in general practice: does detection or disclosure make a difference? *British Medical Journal* 311, pp 1274–1276.

Eastwood P 1995. Promoting peer group support with postnatally depressed women. *Health Visitor* 68(4), pp 148–150.

Effective Health Care 1993. The treatment of depression in primary care. March No. 5.

Eisenberg L 1992. Treating Depression and Anxiety in Primary Care. Closing the Gap Between Knowledge and Practice. *New England Journal of Medicine* 326, pp 1080–1084.

Eli Lilley Centre (nd). *Management of Depression in General Practice*. Eli Lilley Centre, Leicester

Faravelli C, Webb T, Ambonetti A, Fonnesu F and Sessargo A 1985. Prevalence of traumatic early life events in 31 agoraphobic patients with panic attacks. *American Journal of Psychiatry* 142, pp 1493–1494.

Foyster L 1995. Supporting mothers: an inter-disciplinary approach. *Health Visitor* 68(4), pp 151–152.

France R and Robson M 1986. *Behaviour Therapy in Primary Care: A Practical Guide*. London and Sydney: Croom Helm.

Free ML, Oei TPS 1989. Biological and psychological processes in the treatment and maintenance of depression. *Clinical Psychology Review* 9, pp 653–688.

Freeling P, Rao BM, Paykel ES *et al.* 1985. Unrecognised depression in general practice. *British Medical Journal* 290, pp 1880–1883.

Freemantle *et al.* 1994. Prescribing selective serotonin reuptake inhibitors as a strategy for the prevention of suicide. *British Medical Journal* 309, pp 249–253.

Gabe J, Williams P 1987. Is space bad for your health? The relationship between crowding in the home and emotional distress in women. *International Journal of Health Service Research* 17, pp 667–669.

Gillam S 1994. The use of benefits programmes in community health care settings. *Primary Care Management* Vol. 4 No. 1, pp 8–9.

Goldberg D and Huxley P 1992. *Common Mental Disorders: A bio-social model*. Routledge.

Goldberg D, Benjamin S and Creed F 1994. *Psychiatry in General Practice*. Routledge.

Goldberg R J, Novack D H, Gask L 1992. The Recognition and Management of Somatization. What is Needed in Primary Care Training. *Psychosomatics* 33, pp 55–61.

Goldstein RB, Black DW, Nasrallah A and Winokur G 1991. The prediction of suicide: sensitivity, specificity and predictive value of a multivariate model applied to suicide among 1906 patients with affective disorders. *Archives of General Psychiatry* 48, pp 418–422.

Good MJD, Good BJ, Cleary PD 1987. Do patient attitudes influence physician recognition of psychosocial problems in primary care? *Journal of Family Practice* 25, pp 53–59.

Gournay K and Brooking J 1994. Community psychiatric nurses in primary health care. *British Journal of Psychiatry* 165, pp 231–237.

Gunnell D and Frankel S 1994. Prevention of suicide: aspirations and evidence. *British Medical Journal* Vol. 308 May, pp 1227–1233.

The Health of the Nation 1991. London: HMSO.

Hill RG and Shepherd G 1996. Manic depression and the role of the mental health nurse. *Mental Health Nursing* 16(1), pp 18–20.

Hooper PD 1990. Psychological sequelae of sexual abuse in childhood. *British Journal of General Practice* 40, pp 29–31.

Huppert FA, Roth M, Gore M 1987. *Health and Lifestyle Survey, preliminary report.* London: Health Promotion Research Trust.

Irving J, Heath V 1989. *Counselling in General Practice: A guide for general practitioners.* London: British Association for Counselling.

Isacsson G, Holmgren P, Wasserman D, Bergman U 1994. Use of antidepressants among people committing suicide in Sweden. *British Medical Journal* Vol. 308 February, pp 506–509.

Jenkins R, Newton J, Young R 1992. *The Prevention of Depression and Anxiety: The Role of the Primary Care Team.* London: HMSO.

Johnson G *et al.* 1995. Psychiatric comorbidity, health status and functional impairment associated with alcohol misuse and dependence in primary care patients: findings of the PRIME MD–1000 study. *Journal of Consulting and Clinical Psychology* 63(1), pp 133–140.

Johnstone A, Goldberg D 1976. Psychiatric screening in general practice: a controlled trial. *Lancet* 1, pp 605–608.

Jones A, Watts T and Romain S 1995. Facilitating peer group pressure. *Health Visitor* 68(4), p 153.

Karlsson H, Lehtinen V and Joukamaa M 1995. Psychiatric morbidity among frequent attender patients in primary care. *General Hospital Psychiatry* 17, pp 1902–5.

Katon W *et al.* 1995. Collaborative management to achieve treatment guidelines. *JAMA* 273(13), pp 1026–1031.

Kendrick T, BurnsT and Freeling P 1995. Randomised controlled trial of teaching general practitioners to carry out structured assessments of their long term mentally ill patients. *British Medical Journal* 311, pp 93–98.

Kerr M, Blizard R and Mann A 1995. General practitioners and psychiatrists: comparison of attitudes to depression using the depression attitude questionnaire. *British Journal of General Practice* 45, pp 89–92.

Kessler R and Neighbours HW 1986. A new perspective on the relationships among race, social class and psychological distress. *Journal Health Social Behaviour* 27, pp 107–115.

King's Fund 1994. *Community-Oriented Primary Care: A resource for developers.* London: King's Fund.

Ley 1988. *Communicating with Patients.* Chapman & Hall.

Livingstone G, Hawkins A, Graham N et al. 1990. The Gospel Oak study: prevalence rates of dementia, depression and activity rates among elderly residents in inner London. *Psychological Medicine* 20, pp 881–892.

Lloyd K 1992. Ethnicity, primary care and non-psychotic disorders. *International Review of Psychiatry* 4, pp 257–266.

Lloyd K and Jenkins R 1994. In: Paykel E and Jenkins R. *Prevention in Psychiatry.* Chapter 19. London: Gaskell.

Lloyd K and Jenkins 1995a. The economics of depression: department of health initiative in primary care. *British Journal of Psychiatry* (In press).

Lloyd K and Jenkins 1995b. Chronic anxiety and depression in primary care. *Advances in Psychiatric Treatment.* (In press).

Lloyd KR, Jenkins R and Mann A 1996. Long term outcome of patients with neurotic illness in general practice. *British Medical Journal* 313, pp 26–28.

Long CG and Bourne V 1987. Linking professional and self-help resources for anxiety management: a community project. *Journal of the Royal College of General Practitioners* May, pp 199–201.

Lowry S 1990. Housing and health: families and flats. *British Medical Journal* 300, pp 245–247.

Matthews K, Milne S and Ashcroft GW 1994. Role of doctors in the prevention of suicide: the final consultation. *British Journal of General Practice* August, pp 345–348.

May A 1995. Using exercises to tackle postnatal depression. *Health Visitor* 68(4), pp 146–147.

McClarey M and Stokoe B 1995. A multi-disciplinary approach to postnatal depression. *Health Visitor* 68(4), pp 141–143.

Mead M 1995. SSRIs: mood change. *Practice Nurse* February, pp 699–700.

Mental Health Foundation 1995. *Making Life Better: Mental health of older people*. Mental Health Foundation.

Milne D and Covitz F 1988. A comparative evaluation of anxiety management materials in general practice. *Health Education Journal* Vol. 47, No. 2/3, pp 67–69.

Myners-Wallis LM, Gath GH, Lloyd-Harris AR and Tomlinson D 1995. Randomised controlled trial comparing problem-solving treatment and amytrypilene and placebo for major depression in primary care. *British Medical Journal* 310, pp 441–445.

Nietzel MT, Russell RL, Hemmings KA, Gretter ML 1988. Clinical significance of psychotherapy for unipolar depression: a meta-analytical approach to social comparison. *Journal Consultant Clinical Psychology* 55, pp 156–161.

Olfson M *et al*. 1995. The SDDS-PC: A mental aid for multiple mental disorders in primary care. *Psychopharmacology Bulletin* 31(2), pp 415–420.

Painter A 1995. Health visitor identification of postnatal depression. *Health Visitor* 68(4), pp 138–140.

Paris JAG and Player D 1993. Citizens' advice in general practice. *British Medical Journal* Vol. 306 June, pp 1518–1520.

Paykel ES and Priest RG 1992. Recognition and management of depression in general practice: consensus statement. *British Medical Journal* Vol. 305. p 1200.

Pitts F 1995. Comrades in adversity: the group approach. *Health Visitor* 68(4), pp 144–145.

Rand E, Badger L, Coggins D 1988. Towards a resolution of contradictions: utility of feedback from GHQ. *General Hospital Psychiatry* 10, pp189–196.

Richards JP 1990. Postnatal depression: a review of the literature. *British Journal of General Practice* 40, pp 472–476

Robson M 1992. Counselling in general practice A: Options for action: clinical psychology. In: Jenkins R, Newton J and Young R. *The Prevention of Depression and Anxiety*. London: HMSO.

The Royal College of Psychiatrists and The Royal College of General Practitioners (nd). *Shared care of patients with mental health problems*. The Royal College of General Practitioners.

Rutz W, Von Knorring L, Walinder J 1992. Long Term Effects of an Educational Program for General Practitioners Given by the Swedish Committee for the Prevention and Treatment of Depression. *Acta Psychiatr Scand* 85, pp 83–88.

Saunders P 1995. Depression in life-threatening illness and its treatment. *Nursing Times* 91(11), pp 41–43.

Scott J, Eccleston D and Boys R 1992. Can we predict the persistence of depression? *British Journal of Psychiatry* 161, pp 633–7.

Sharp D 1992. Liaison between providers of primary care: early detection difficulties B: Predicting postnatal depression. In: Jenkins R, Newton J and Young R. *The Prevention of Depression and Anxiety*. London: HMSO.

Sheldon M 1992. *Counselling in General Practice*. RCGP.

Silver FW and Ruckle JL 1989. Depression management techniques in primary care. *Postgraduate Medicine* Vol. 85, No. 4, pp 359–366.

Smeeton N, Wilkinson G, Skuse D, Fry J 1992. A longitudinal study of general practitioner consultations for psychiatric disorder in adolescence. *Psychological Medicine* 22, pp 495–502.

Smith ML, Glass G 1977. Meta-analysis of psychotherapy. *American Psychology* 32, p 9.

Sorby NGD, Reavley W, Huber JW 1991. Self help programme for anxiety in general practice: controlled trial of an anxiety management booklet. *British Journal of General Practice* October, pp 417–420.

Thompson D 1993. *Mental Illness: The fundamental facts*. Mental Health Foundation.

Tylee AT, Freeling P and Kerry S 1993. Why do general practitioners recognise major depression in one woman patient yet miss it in another? *British Journal of General Practice* 43, pp 327–330.

US Department of Health and Human Services 1993. *Depression in Primary Care. Volume 1 Detection and Diagnosis*. US Department of Health and Human Services.

Üstün TB and Sartorius N (eds) 1995. *Mental Illness in General Health Care*. Chichester: John Wiley.

Üstün TB *et al*. 1995. New classification for mental disorders with management guidelines for use in primary care: ICD–10 PHC. Chapter 5. *British Journal of General Practice* 45, pp 211–215.

van den Brink W, Leenstra A, Ormel J, van den Willige G 1991. Mental health intervention programs in primary care: their scientific basis. *Journal of Affective Disorders* 21, 273–284.

van Marwijk HWJ et al 1995. Evaluation of the feasibility, reliability and diagnostic value of shortened versions of the geriatric depression scale. *British Journal of General Practice* 45, pp 195–199.

Vassilas, CA and Morgan HG 1993. General practitioners' contact with victims of suicide. *British Medical Journal* 307, pp 300–301.

Vázquez-Barquero JL, Diez-Manrique JF, Gaite L, Iglesias García C, Artal J, Roberts SE and Wilkinson G 1992. Why people with probable minor psychiatric morbidity consult a doctor. *Psychological Medicine* 22, pp 495–502.

Wilkinson DG 1989. *Depression: Recognition and treatment in general practice*. Oxford: Radcliffe Medical Press.

Wilkinson G 1992. The role of the practice nurse in the management of depression. *International Review of Psychiatry* Vol. 4, No. 3/4, pp 311–315.

Wilkinson G 1992a. *Anxiety: Recognition and treatment in general practice*. Oxford: Radcliffe Medical Press.

Williams D 1996. Bringing depression out into the open. *Healthlines* February, pp 20–21.

Wright AF, Perini AF 1987. Hidden psychiatric illness: use of the general health questionnaire in general practice. *Journal of the Royal College of General Practice* 37, pp 164–167.

Zung L, Magill M, Moore J 1983. Recognition and treatment of depression in a family medical practice. *Journal of Clinical Psychiatry* 4, pp 1–9.

Further reading

The following titles are particularly relevant in the design of COPC interventions, although none makes specific references to the COPC methodology.

Armstrong E 1995. *Mental Health Issues in Primary Care*. Houndmills: Macmillan.

France R and Robson M 1986. *Behaviour Therapy in Primary Care: A practical guide*. London and Sydney: Croom Helm.

Goldberg D and Huxley P 1992. *Common Mental Disorders: A bio-social model*. Routledge.

Goldberg D, Benjamin S and Creed F 1994. *Psychiatry in General Practice*. Routledge.

Jenkins R, Newton J, Young R 1992. *The Prevention of Depression and Anxiety: The role of the primary care team*. London: HMSO.

Kendrick, Tylee and Freely 1996. *Prevention of Mental Illness in General Practice*.

King's Fund 1994. *Community-Oriented Primary Care: A resource for developers*. London: King's Fund.

Paykel ES ed 1992. *Handbook of Affective Disorders*. Churchill Livingstone 2nd ed.

US Department of Health and Human Services 1993. *Depression in Primary Care. Volume 1 Detection and Diagnosis*. US Department of Health and Human Services.

Wilkinson G 1989. *Depression: Recognition and treatment in general practice*. Oxford: Radcliffe Medical Press.

Wilkinson G 1992. *Anxiety: Recognition and treatment in general practice*. Oxford: Radcliffe Medical Press.

Appendix 1

Edinburgh Postnatal Depression Scale[*]

The Edinburgh Postnatal Depression Scale (EPDS) has been developed to assist primary care health professionals to detect mothers suffering from postnatal depression; a distressing disorder more prolonged than the 'blues' (which occur in the first week after delivery) but less severe than puerperal psychosis.

Previous studies have shown that postnatal depression affects at least 10 per cent of women and that many depressed mothers remain untreated. These mothers may cope with their baby and with household tasks, but their enjoyment of life is seriously affected and it is possible that there are long-term effects on the family.

The EPDS was developed at health centres in Livingston and Edinburgh. It consists of ten short statements. The mother underlines which of the four possible responses is closest to how she has been feeling during the past week. Most mothers complete the scale without difficulty in less than 5 minutes.

The validation study showed that mothers who scored above a threshold 12/13 were likely to be suffering from a depressive illness of varying severity. Nevertheless the EPDS score should *not* override clinical judgement. A careful clinical assessment should be carried out to confirm the diagnosis. The scale indicates how the mother has felt *during the previous week*, and in doubtful cases it may be usefully repeated after 2 weeks. The scale will not detect mothers with anxiety neuroses, phobias or personality disorders.

Instructions for users

1. The mother is asked to underline the response which comes closest to how she has been feeling in the previous 7 days.
2. All ten items must be completed.

---

*Reproduced by kind permission from Cox *et al*. (1987).

3. Care should be taken to avoid the possibility of the mother discussing her answers with others.
4. The mother should complete the scale herself, unless she has limited English or has difficulty with reading.
5. The EPDS may be used at 6–8 weeks to screen postnatal women. The child health clinic, postnatal check-up or a home visit may provide suitable opportunities for its completion.

EDINBURGH POSTNATAL DEPRESSION SCALE (EPDS)
J.L. Cox, J.M. Holden, R. Sagovsky
Department of Psychiatry, University of Edinburgh

Name:
Address:
Baby's age:

As you have recently had a baby, we would like to know how you are feeling. Please UNDERLINE the answer which comes closest to how you have felt IN THE PAST 7 DAYS, not just how you feel today.

Here is an example, already completed.

I have felt happy:
 Yes, all the time
 <u>Yes, most of the time</u>
 No, not very often
 No, not at all

This would mean: 'I have felt happy most of the time' during the past week. Please complete the other questions in the same way.

In the past 7 days:

1. I have been able to laugh and see the funny side of things
 As much as I always could
 Not quite so much now
 Definitely not so much now
 Not at all

2. I have looked forward with enjoyment to things
 As much as I ever did
 Rather less than I used to
 Definitely less than I used to
 Hardly at all

*3. I have blamed myself unnecessarily when things went wrong
 Yes, most of the time
 Yes, some of the time
 Not very often
 No, never

cont.

4. I have been anxious or worried for no good reason
    No, not at all
    Hardly ever
    Yes, sometimes
    Yes, very often

*5. I have felt scared or panicky for no very good reason
    Yes, quite a lot
    Yes, sometimes
    No, not much
    No, not at all

*6. Things have been getting on top of me
    Yes, most of the time I haven't been able to cope at all
    Yes, sometimes I haven't been coping as well as usual
    No, most of the time I have coped quite well
    No, I have been coping as well as ever

*7. I have been so unhappy that I have had difficulty sleeping
    Yes, most of the time
    Yes, sometimes
    Not very often
    No, not at all

*8. I have felt sad or miserable
    Yes, most of the time
    Yes, quite often
    Not very often
    No, not at all

*9. I have been so unhappy that I have been crying
    Yes, most of the time
    Yes, quite often
    Only occasionally
    No, never

*10. The thought of harming myself has occurred to me
    Yes, quite often
    Sometimes
    Hardly ever

Response categories are scored 0, 1, 2 and 3 according to increased severity of the symptom.

Items marked with an asterisk are reverse scored (i.e. 3, 2, 1 and 0). The total score is calculated by adding together the scores for each of the ten items. Users may reproduce the scale without further permission providing they respect copyright (which remains with the *British Journal of Psychiatry*) by quoting the names of the authors, the title and the source of the paper in all reproduced copies.

Marks and Mathews Fear Questionnaire

Name .... Age .... Sex .... Date ....

Choose a number from the scale below to show how much you avoid each of the situations listed, because of fear or other unpleasant feelings. Then write the number you chose in the box opposite each situation.

0	1	2	3	4	5	6	7	8
Would not avoid it		Slightly avoid it		Definitely avoid it		Markedly avoid it		Always avoid it

1. Main phobia you want treated (describe in your own words)

    ....

2. Injections or minor surgery ☐
3. Eating and drinking with other people ☐
4. Hospitals ☐
5. Travelling alone by bus or coach ☐
6. Walking alone in busy streets ☐
7. Being watched or stared at ☐
8. Going into crowded shops ☐
9. Talking to people in authority ☐
10. Sight of blood ☐
11. Being criticised ☐
12. Going alone far from home ☐
13. Thought of injury or illness ☐
14. Speaking or acting to an audience ☐
15. Large open spaces ☐
16. Going to the dentist ☐
17. Other situations (describe)

    ....

Leave blank ☐ ☐ ☐   ☐

Ag Bl Soc TOTAL

(Omit 1 & 17)

Now choose a number from the scale below to show how much you are troubled by each problem listed, and write the number in the box opposite.

0	1	2	3	4	5	6	7	8
Hardly at all		Slightly troublesome		Definitely troublesome		Markedly troublesome		Always troublesome

18. Feeling miserable or depressed ☐
19. Feeling irritable or angry ☐
20. Feeling tense or panicky ☐
21. Upsetting thoughts coming into your mind ☐
22. Feeling you or your surroundings are strange or unreal ☐
23. Other feelings (please describe)

....

TOTAL ☐

How would you state the present state of your phobic symptoms on the scale below?

0	1	2	3	4	5	6	7	8
No phobias present		slightly disturbing not really disabling		definitely disturbing/ disabling		markedly disturbing/ disabling		very severely disturbing/ disabling

Please circle one number between 0 and 8.

Acknowledgement: This scale is reproduced by kind permission of the authors, Professor Isaac Marks and Professor Andrew Mathews. Further information and permission to use and reproduce the scale may be obtained from the authors at The Institute of Psychiatry, De Crespigny Park, London SE5 8AF.

Appendix 3

Self Help for Anxiety*

Anxiety is necessary to help cope with danger or difficulty such as driving in fog or working with dangerous tools. Problems with excess anxiety are, however, very common and about one person in ten consults a doctor about them at some time. Tablets such as tranquillisers are one answer and they do help for a while but gradually they lose effect as you go on taking them. They also may give rise to side-effects when you try to stop them.

What is Anxiety?

It affects both body and mind producing worrying feelings of fear and apprehension together with physical feelings of tension, trembling, churning stomach, nausea, diarrhoea, backache and palpitations. These physical symptoms can easily be put down to other worrying causes like cancer or heart attacks – thus increasing fear.

When is Anxiety a Real Problem?

When it interferes with life in the absence of real danger or goes on too long after the danger is past.

Why Does This Happen?

All of us come under stress at some time or another. Some of us feel the effects more than others but even those who become anxious rather easily can learn to cope with it.

What are the Consequences of Persistent Anxiety?

(1) *Upsetting Thoughts* that you may have a serious physical illness or be in real danger increase the feelings:

Bodily feelings ⇌ Anxiety ⇌ Fear of anxiety

(2) *Avoiding Things or Places that Make You Anxious*. It is normal to avoid real danger but anxiety may lead you to avoid things like shops, crowded places and trains which are not really dangerous. At first avoidance makes you feel better but:

*Reproduced by kind permission from France & Robson (1986), pp. 63–66.

(i)   Relief is only temporary – you may worry what will happen next time;

(ii) Every time you avoid something it *is* harder next time you try to face it;

(iii) Gradually you want to avoid more and more things.

(3) Loss of Confidence. Confidence is built up by doing things successfully. If you find that you can no longer do things that you used to do successfully, confidence is lost and can only be regained by building gradually from tackling the easiest tasks first.

REMEMBER   (i) Anxiety does produce physical symptoms like rapid heart rate but it does not produce physical harm like heart attacks.

(ii) It makes you tired by using energy uselessly but does not cause nervous breakdowns.

Controlling Symptoms

Many people already know some ways of making their symptoms better and some things which make them worse. Write these down and see if you can use this information to help in other circumstances.

Relaxation

Relaxation can help in relieving uncomfortable muscular tension, tiredness and worry. It also helps to slow down the speeding up and mental wheelspin which occur with anxiety.

Tape recorded instructions show you first how to relax your whole body, then how you can do it quickly in a number of different situations and finally how to use it to cope with the onset of feelings and anxiety or tension. The exercises teach you what it feels like to be totally relaxed and where your particular centres of tension are.

Regular practice is essential and should be at a settled time of day which is reserved for it. When you have completed the relaxation exercises try to imagine yourself in a situation where you have felt perfectly calm and contented. Re-create the sights and sounds of that situation in your mind. A list of relaxing situations such as good days in the country or on holiday is useful for this purpose.

Start to use relaxation in circumstances when you are beginning to feel anxious – good exercises for this purpose are relaxing the brows and neck, dropping the shoulders and practising slow, regular shallow breathing. A key word like 'calm' or 'relax' can be used to start the sequence. Physical exercise like jogging, cycling, swimming or playing a ball game may also help to relieve symptoms.

Rapid Anxious Breathing

Such breathing can make you tremble, feel dizzy, produce a thumping heart and give you a tingling sensation in your hands and feet. This can be very worrying and give you the idea that you may be having a serious illness like a stroke or heart attack. These symptoms can be quickly controlled by slow, shallow breathing at the rate of 8–12 breaths per minute.

Rushing and Posture

Plan your timetable in advance in order to avoid rushing. You will probably find that you get just as much done. When you have finished or are having a planned break, sit in a comfortable relaxed posture – not hunched on the edge of your chair.

Distraction

Tense, worrying thoughts tend to produce a vicious circle. Try to turn your attention off these thoughts and fill your mind with something else – for example:

(i) Concentrating on what is going on around you. According to where you are you can try counting the branches on a tree, the cars in the street or the soup tins in a stack. There are many possible variations on this theme.
(ii) Mental activity such as remembering a list, or a poem or doing mental arithmetic.
(iii) Physical activity such as walking, gardening or ironing.

Controlling Upsetting Thoughts

Half-formed upsetting thoughts and images can make you feel anxious or keep anxiety going. The thought that the sharp pain in your chest may be due to a heart attack makes the pain more sinister and threatening.

It is important first to study your thinking and find out exactly what your upsetting thoughts are. This is quite difficult because they are automatic and come and go very quickly so that initially you may not be aware of them and need to practise hard in order to identify them. Try to write them down exactly as they occur when you feel tense. They may be quite simple like 'Here we go again' or 'This is the way it started last time'. Once you know what you are thinking you can examine the thoughts carefully and identify those that are exaggerated or unrealistic. 'I didn't get the job so perhaps nobody will employ me', 'l feel tense about talking at the meeting which shows I shall make a hash of it' or 'I punished William unfairly so I am a lousy mother'. There are positive and more reasonable alternatives to all these thoughts. Try to write them down and then look at some of your own thoughts and try to find more reasonable alternatives. This is quite difficult at first but with practice, and sometimes a bit of help, it gets easier.

Dealing with Avoidance and Loss of Confidence

Avoidance easily builds up with anxiety and makes things harder. It is countered by gradually getting back into the habit of doing things which build up confidence. The steps are as follows:

(1) Make a list of the situations that you avoid or that make you anxious.
(2) Arrange these in order according to how difficult it would be for you to face each one.
(3) Select the easiest item on the list as the first target when you start to practise.
(4) Make yourself repeat this item many times until you can do it without difficulty.
(5) Then move on to the next item on the list and so on until you are able to tackle the whole list.

Remember that to be helpful, practice must be regular, frequent and prolonged.

Our thanks are due to Ms Gillian Butler and the Dept of Psychiatry, Oxford University, for their permission to use much of the material on this advice sheet.